# Can I Eat That?

A nutritional guide through the
dietary maze for Type 2 diabetics

## Jenefer Roberts

ROBINSON

ROBINSON

First published in Great Britain in 2016 by Robinson

1 3 5 7 9 10 8 6 4 2

**Important note:**
This book is not intended as a substitute for medical advice or treatment. Any
person with a condition requiring medical attention should consult a qualified
medical practitioner or suitable therapist.

A CIP catalogue record for this book is available from the British Library.

ISBN: 978-1-47213-630-5 (paperback)

Typeset by Mousemat Design Limited
Printed and bound by CPI Group (UK) Ltd, Croydon, CR0 4YY

Papers used by Robinson are from well-managed forests and other responsible
sources.

Robinson
is an imprint of Little, Brown Book Group
Carmelite House, 50 Victoria Embankment, London EC4Y 0DZ

An Hachette UK Company
www.hachette.co.uk

www.littlebrown.co.uk

To Peter,
without whom this book would not have happened,
thank you

# Table of Contents

# Introduction

This book was started in a fit of exasperation. Newly diagnosed with Type 2 diabetes, my husband was constantly asking if the things he fancied were okay to eat. In supermarkets, cafés and restaurants he would enquire, 'Can I eat that?' and when the answer was no, the supplementary question was, 'Why not?' He read the leaflets and books but switched off – the technical bits were boring, he said – and I found myself getting annoyed. So I started to write it all down for him. These notes turned into a book and when it was finished it seemed a good idea to include some recipes.

Husband Peter had suddenly started to drink and pee a lot so we knew that something was wrong. Sure enough, a few days later he came back from the doctor with the diagnosis of Type 2 diabetes. 'It could have been something much worse,' I told him, but he was very upset and went into a state of shock for a week. He told everyone he was dying and was too frightened to eat anything. This was understandable as he was a man who had been fit, healthy and active for six decades. He walked four dogs regularly and visits to the doctor's surgery had been infrequent.During the next three weeks Peter, an enthusiastic follower of the pork pie and pizza diet, lived largely on fruit. Everything else frightened him and because he had cut out all the foods he loved we anticipated a greatly improved blood-glucose-level reading at his next appointment. So it was a shock when it was found to be little changed and the diabetes nurse shook her head and explained that a diet containing large amounts of fruit was almost as bad for him as his previous diet had been. 'Eat more vegetables,' she said.

That sounded straightforward enough. We liked vegetables so I thought that most of the meals we enjoyed could remain on the menu. Cottage pie with its potato topping, tomato pizzas with a little cheese on top, baked potatoes with a healthy prawn or coleslaw topping, these would all be fine. However, a few days later, after reading information sheets and a book on diabetes, I had to revise my opinions. I had learnt that Type 2 diabetes always has the potential to turn into something 'much worse' and that things called GI values are of particular importance to people with the condition.

The initials GI stand for glycaemic index. This measurement is the rate at which, after eating, carbohydrates in food are turned into bloodstream glucose. People with diabetes need to eat foods that have a 'slow burn' and this means foods with a low GI value. The foods which featured regularly in our diet included potatoes, pizza, parsnips and pastry. These, I discovered, all have high GI values and now had to be avoided.

This was worrying and confusing. I no longer knew what to cook, or how to cook it. GI values were a puzzle and an approach based on common sense just did not work. Surely mashed potatoes would be a healthier option than chips? Not necessarily so.

For the first month or so after Peter was diagnosed I cooked meals using ingredients that had a low GI value without any real understanding of what I was doing. But I knew that the return of a healthy husband depended upon a different style of cooking. So sugar and refined white flour were banned from the kitchen and for a while there was no more cake or biscuit making, no more pastry-based meals and no potatoes. Rice, pasta, pizzas and white bread became a hazy memory. Allowed were (to us) freaky things like beans, pulses and lentils and boring but wholesome things like broccoli and granary bread. Living on food like this was not an appealing prospect and I slightly resented this change in our shopping and eating habits. But there seemed no alternative and a little book containing the GI values of hundreds of foods became my constant companion. It was consulted in the kitchen when cooking, in the supermarket when shopping and in the café or restaurant on the few occasions that we dared to eat out.

And so began our new life as shopping and cooking styles underwent a revolution. Supermarket trolley jams were caused as we struggled with the microscopic print on food labels. Many items previously tossed light-heartedly into the trolley were excluded. Alternative recipes for favourite meals were discovered, many sourced online (indeed the internet has low-GI alternatives for almost every dish imaginable. I tested many of them. Some tasted good; quite a lot were offered to the dog and rejected.)

Cooking now takes longer. More vegetables have to be prepared. Beans and pulses tend to be bland so a greater variety and quantity of herbs and spices are needed. And, of course, the GI value of a food or a meal is not its full story. Crisps, cream and chocolate all have low GIs!

Learning to cope with a diagnosis of diabetes is not easy. It is an insidious condition – often there are no definitive answers to questions concerning diet and a person can continue to eat foods that he or she shouldn't, without any immediate effect. The food does not make them feel unwell and the danger exists of a slow shift back to unhealthy eating habits. We have talked with health professionals, read books and researched the internet. Conflicting advice has frequently puzzled us but has also been the motivation to dig deeper into the subject, and the result has been the rediscovery of some of the things we probably learnt at school but have long forgotten. We hope that sharing this knowledge will help others.

An important discovery is that food that is good for people with diabetes is food that is good for everyone. A diet that is restricted (the pessimistic view) or *different but better* (the optimistic view) will become a necessity, but people with Type 2 diabetes can still enjoy wining and dining.

This book starts with the basic facts of nutrition. This is because books and leaflets about diabetes all use words like carbohydrates, sugars, glucose and digestion. Most people have some idea of what these words mean, but a deeper knowledge will help them to understand the diabetic condition. Sections on food and diet follow and these may reveal surprising facts about our everyday food. A recipe section follows.

Cup measures are US cup size (8 fluid ounces). A Tala Cook's Measure will help you calculate the correct quantity if you don't have US cups.

We hope that the references to research and competing theories about food, nutrition and health will interest readers and encourage them to read further. Like us, they may discover some interesting discrepancies between what we know about our food and the advice we receive.

# Abbreviations

CHO    Carbohydrate
EFA    Essential fatty acid
FDA    Food and Drug Administration; the US agency
       responsible for the safety of drugs and food
FSA    Food Standards Agency; a UK independent
       government department responsible for food safety
       and hygiene
GDA    Guideline daily amount
MUFA  Monounsaturated fatty acid
PUFA   Polyunsaturated fatty acid

# 1

# What is Diabetes?

Once upon a time people with Type 2 diabetes were advised to cut down on sugary things like cake, biscuits and ice-cream and satisfy their appetite with savoury food like bread and potatoes. It was generally understood that if people followed this advice their blood glucose levels would remain under control. But in the 1980s a Canadian professor discovered that bread and potatoes actually caused blood glucose levels to increase quite dramatically only a short period after being eaten. This came as a surprise and it was after this discovery that the glycaemic index, showing values for different foods, began to be compiled.

When a person eats, their digestive system breaks the food down into a sugar called glucose which enters the bloodstream. This causes a rise in blood glucose levels and this in turn triggers the release of insulin – the hormone which is needed to convert this blood glucose into energy. Any excess that is not used as energy is stored as fat.

People with *Type 1 diabetes* cannot produce any insulin so their blood glucose levels remain high. They need insulin injections.

People with *Type 2 diabetes* either cannot produce enough insulin or they have 'insulin resistance' meaning they cannot use it efficiently (see 'What is Insulin Resistance?' in Appendix 1). In both cases they cannot convert all of their blood glucose into energy and so their blood glucose levels remain higher than normal. Persistently high or fluctuating levels of blood glucose are dangerous as they inflict hidden damage to the body. Type 2 diabetes can sometimes be controlled through exercise and diet, the advice about diet being to eat foods that do not convert too quickly into glucose. But identifying these foods is not straightforward, as the following extract from the blog of a highly exasperated Type 2 diabetic illustrates:

> So, you've just been diagnosed with type 2 diabetes. Obviously, your first question is, 'Holy crap, is this gonna kill me?' The answer is, well, maybe . . . or maybe not . . . probably not . . . but then again . . . depends on what you eat. If you eat the wrong things it can get worse . . . or maybe not . . . Trying to figure out what you can eat is a bitch. One way is to pretend you're a rabbit and go with your instincts. If you're not sure what a rabbit eats, follow one around for a few days and when they start to eat something take it away from them and eat it. Oh! Except carrots. You can't eat carrots . . . well, maybe you can – maybe not . . . Actually, there are a few things you can eat. A quick web search will turn up tons of T2 diabetic-friendly recipes for delicious meals requiring only a total of 4 or 5 hours preparation time by somebody who doesn't have anything else to do but cook all day (if you like things like Curried Flax Patties) . . .
>
> (www.digitalbirdcrap.com/diabetes)

When we tried to find out what a person with Type 2 diabetes *should* eat we read books, asked health professionals, read the leaflets they gave us and still could not answer this question to our total satisfaction. But this was partly because we did not know enough about basic nutrition, so we found out some of the things a person newly diagnosed with diabetes really *does* need to know about food.

## 2

# Things You Need to Know about Food

Food gives us energy and lets us grow. It is made up of energy-giving and body-building nutrients and the big three are proteins, carbohydrates and fats. Other nutrients include vitamins and minerals. Food made from plants also contains fibre.

To understand diabetes it helps to know a little about what happens to food when it is eaten, so we shall follow the journey of a cheese and tomato sandwich – a nicely balanced little meal containing carbohydrate, protein, fat and fibre, distributed in varying proportions between the bread, cheese and tomato.

After the first bite, enzymes in mouth saliva immediately start to digest certain types of starch (carbohydrate) in the food and turn it into sugars. The masticated food then enters the stomach. Here other enzymes also get to work digesting the fats and proteins in the food. After this, the semi-digested food moves through to the small intestine, where further absorption of nutrients occurs. What is left then enters the large intestine (colon) where fermentation occurs. What remains then enters the rectum, where it is stored until a visit is made to the smallest room.

This brief description shows how nutrients in a meal are processed in different parts of the digestive system at different time intervals after being eaten. **This is key to understanding why some foods have a high glycaemic index value and other foods have a low value.**

The diet we eat consists of a mixture of foods. A good diet will provide adequate amounts of all the nutrients from a wide range of food. Macronutrients are the nutrients we need in large amounts. Micronutrients are the nutrients we need in small amounts.

*There are three macronutrients.* They are:

• *Protein*, which provides material (amino acids) for growth and repair. They can be converted to carbohydrate and used to provide energy (4 kilocalories per gram).

• *Carbohydrates*, which provide the body with energy and may also be converted into body fat (4 kilocalories per gram).

• *Fats*, which provide energy in a more concentrated form than carbohydrates. Fat is also an important component of cells within the body, which is why everyone needs some fat in their diet (9 kilocalories per gram). The figures show just how high in calories fat is compared to protein and carbohydrates.

*There are two micronutrients.* They are:

• *Minerals*, which are used in growth and repair and help to regulate body processes.

• *Vitamins*, which help to regulate body processes.

## PROTEIN

Protein is found in meat, fish, dairy products, cereals, eggs, grains and nuts. It is made up of amino acids, eight of which our bodies are unable to make and are therefore described as 'essential' (see 'What is Protein?' in Appendix 1). Protein is often seen as the good guy of the big three, as the other two may make you fat or ill. And protein is relatively uncomplicated for people with diabetes. They can eat it! The recommended daily requirement for an adult human is surprisingly modest, being 0.8g of protein per 1 kilogram of body weight. Most people eat more protein than they actually need. Protein is more complicated for vegetarians as they have to combine certain foods in order to receive all eight essential amino acids.

## CARBOHYDRATES

Carbohydrates are sugars and starches. The human body needs carbohydrates to make glucose – our main source of energy.

Starches and sugars vary in the amount of time they take to be digested. *Rapidly Digested Starch* breaks down quickly into simple sugars. Carbohydrates with a lot of this type of starch (e.g. large potatoes) have a high glycaemic index – they cause blood glucose to rise quickly and stay high for longer. People with Type 2 diabetes often refer to these sudden elevated levels of blood glucose as sugar spikes. In comparison, *Slowly Digested Starch* breaks down in the small intestine up to two hours after being eaten. Carbohydrates containing a lot of this type of starch have a low glycaemic index – they do not cause sugar spikes. The starch in beans is a combination of this and another type, called resistant starch, which takes even longer to be digested.

*Resistant Starch* gets as far as the large intestine (colon) without being broken down into any sugars at all and when it reaches the colon it is fermented by colon bacteria. The beneficial effect of this type of starch even includes lowering the glycaemic response to carbohydrates that are eaten later. This is known as the 'second meal effect'. (There will be more about this later.)

### What happens next?

We have seen that some types of carbohydrate are digested very quickly. These, the ones that break down rapidly into glucose, trigger a large release of insulin from the pancreas. Insulin causes the glucose to be stored in the cells as glycogen, but this rapid conversion causes levels of blood glucose to drop, and this can leave a person feeling tired and hungry. They may then be tempted to eat again. People who become locked into this cycle of hunger and eating are likely to gain weight.

---

**CARBOHYDRATES: SUMMARY**

We need carbohydrates to make glucose, which is our main source of energy.
Carbohydrates are found in sugars and starches. The body turns these into glucose.
Some carbohydrates (e.g. white flour, table sugar) are turned into glucose very quickly.
Some carbohydrates take much longer to be turned into glucose.
A release of insulin is needed to turn blood glucose into energy or, if unused, into fat.

---

## FATS

Fats, our third main nutrient, are now commonly associated with hamburgers, chips, butter and heart attacks. 'Sugar and fat are equally bad,' said the dietitian when, a few years ago, Peter asked her which was worse, and her doom-laden words – 'equally bad' – stuck in the memory. We went home and threw away all the cheese and butter in the fridge!

But fat is tricky. There are conflicting theories as to which are the good and which are the bad fats and it is difficult for non-scientific people to sort out the facts from the vast amount of chat about it all. Perhaps the situation is best summed up like this. We know what fat is. We are not so certain about what it does to us.

So what is it? Fat is made up of different kinds of fatty acids – chains of carbon, some bonding with a lot of hydrogen atoms, some with only one or a few. *Saturated fat* contains the maximum number of hydrogen bonds possible. It is, literally, saturated with hydrogen. *Unsaturated fat* contains one (*monounsaturated*) or many (*polyunsaturated*) hydrogen bonds. Foods contain different proportions of saturated and unsaturated fat. As we have seen, the difference between them lies in their chemical structure and is the reason why a packet of butter is solid and a bottle of vegetable oil is liquid.

Fats from animal sources (and coconut and palm oils) contain a high proportion of saturated fat. Saturated fats are solid at room temperature.

Fats from vegetables, fish and nuts contain a high proportion of unsaturated fats. Two important types are *monounsaturated* and *polyunsaturated fat*. Again, the difference between them lies in their chemical structure. Unsaturated fats are liquid at room temperature. Omega-3 and omega-6 are types of polyunsaturated fatty acids.

*Trans fats* are vegetable oils that have been hydrogenated to make them solid. Liquid vegetable oil is chemically processed and packed with hydrogen atoms, which converts the oil to a solid. Hydrogenation was seized upon by the food industry as it prolongs the shelf life of products, gives food a nice texture and makes oil reusable in deep-fat frying. However, consumption of trans fat is now linked to heart disease and its use in processed food is less widespread. The labelling of trans fats on processed food items is now compulsory.

**The conventional view about which fats are good for us**
The conventional view is that saturated fat is harmful to health. The fat comes mainly from animal sources, as does cholesterol, a waxy fat-like substance. Both are linked to heart disease. As food that contains saturated fat is also likely to contain cholesterol, the advice has been to cut back on both. A diet high in saturated fat and cholesterol was thought to raise blood cholesterol levels and be a major cause of ill-health.

The beneficial fats were thought to be the monounsaturated and polyunsaturated fats. These are found in a variety of foods and particularly in plant-related food. These fats can actually lower blood cholesterol levels. They therefore make a positive contribution to good health.

This has been the accepted view for the last fifty years or so and most people took heed. They stopped eating cheese and eggs.

They swapped butter for margarine and full-fat milk for skimmed milk. They felt guilty about the occasional indulgence of a fried breakfast. Over this period the consumption of processed vegetable oils increased two- to fourfold. Yet rates of heart disease, cancer and diabetes continued to increase and this has led writers to question the accepted view.

Mary G. Enig is the nutritional researcher who, in the 1970s, first established the danger of trans fat. She also pointed out that reducing the consumption of saturated fat was not reducing the risk of heart disease, cancer or weight gain in Western society. Her argument was that the saturated fat that occurs naturally in dairy and coconut products satisfies hunger and therefore reduces calorie intake (see 'What is a Calorie?' in Appendix 1). She believed that a surfeit of highly processed carbohydrates and polyunsaturated fats – the type found in many margarines and spreads – was more of a health risk than the consumption of butter, cream, milk, cheese and coconut oil, all of which contain additional valuable nutrients.

Argument and counter-argument on the subject of saturated fat continues. Many books and articles have been published and, when considered together, they are frequently convincing, contradictory and confusing, often all at the same time!

### So where are we today?
There is consensus that trans fat is a significant health risk. It increases the levels of bad cholesterol and, simultaneously, lowers the level of good cholesterol in our blood (see 'What is Good Cholesterol? What is Bad Cholesterol?' in Appendix 1).

There is consensus that monounsaturated fats (found in plant foods like nuts, avocados, rapeseed oil, olive oil and also in poultry) have positive health benefits. They can increase good cholesterol and reduce bad cholesterol. Additionally, they contain vitamin E – an important antioxidant.

There may be gradual acceptance that saturated fat is not the health risk it was thought to be a few years ago, but this is not yet reflected in public health or government guidelines.

> In population studies, there is clearly no association of dietary saturated fat and heart disease, yet dietary guidelines advocate its restriction. That's not scientific. But studies measuring saturated fat in the blood and heart disease risks show there is an association. The question is, what causes people to store saturated fat? It is the over-consumption of carbohydrate relative to a person's tolerance that drives accumulation of saturated fat in the body.
>
> (Jeff Volek, Professor of Human Sciences,
> Ohio State University, November 2014)

Dietitians still advise limiting the consumption of all types of fat, as they are heavy on calories. But it is beginning to be understood that the situation is more complex. Although fats are higher in calories than carbohydrates, when eaten they satisfy hunger better. That feeling of fullness, or being satiated, tells us to stop eating.

Professor Volek's advice is that 'it makes more sense to focus on carb restriction than fat restriction'.

### Are polyunsaturated fats now the bad ones?
Some people think so but the evidence is inconclusive. Polyunsaturated fat used to be considered heart healthy and is still considered so by many medical and health authorities – use them in preference to saturated fat they say. But researchers have begun to look more closely at polyunsaturated fat and are highlighting two significant facts:

1.  Polyunsaturated fats are likely to contain high amounts of omega-6 fatty acid but low levels, if any, of omega-3.

2.  Because of its chemical structure, polyunsaturated fat is more

13

prone to oxidisation than saturated or monounsaturated fat. If oxidisation occurs, the fat goes rancid and, when this happens, 'free radicals' are formed. These are harmful chemical compounds that are linked to chronic disease. Some writers claim that seed and vegetable oils, highly processed products, become oxidised by the industrial processes used to manufacture them, and there are now books and websites that will tell you to avoid these highly processed polyunsaturated fats. Sally Fallon, an American nutritionist who worked with Mary G. Enig, writes: 'The cause of heart disease is not animal fats and cholesterol but rather a number of factors inherent in modern diets, including excess consumption of vegetable oils and hydrogenated fats' (Sally Fallon, *Nourishing Traditions*).

---

**FAT: SUMMARY**

Fats are made up of different kinds of fatty acids.

Fat is an essential nutrient required for key body functions. It is also a source of energy. There are different types of fat.

Saturated fat comes mainly from animal products.

There is a statistical but not necessarily causal connection between consumption of saturated fat and ill-health.

On a chemical level saturated fat is saturated (fully bonded) with hydrogen atoms. Saturated fats are solid at room temperature.

Unsaturated fat comes mainly from plant sources and fish.

Unsaturated fats have one (monounsaturated) or many (polyunsaturated) hydrogen bonds. They are liquid at room temperature.

Trans fats are vegetable oils that have been industrially bombarded with hydrogen to make them solid. They are known to be harmful.

Monounsaturated and polyunsaturated fats are promoted as a healthy alternative to saturated fat. Some writers now question whether this is true of the poly fats.

Omega-3 and omega-6 are polyunsaturated essential fatty acids that the body cannot make for itself. Eating food with the right balance between them contributes to good health.

All fats are high in calories.

---

### Essential fatty acids – omega-3 and omega-6

It is probably clear by now that the question 'what is a good fat?' is not so easy to answer. We are now going to confuse matters even further!

Most people know that omega-3 and omega-6, essential fatty acids, are a 'good thing'. They may not know that omega-6 can also be a 'bad thing'. Omega-3 and omega-6 are both essential but one of them may also be contributing to modern chronic disease.

Essential fatty acids are polyunsaturated fats that cannot be produced by the human body but are essential for health and brain function. We require only two: omega-3 and omega-6. There are actually many types of omega-3s and omega-6s. The difference between all of them is down to small but significant chemical differences.

*Omega-3* fatty acids are formed in the green leaves of plants. They are found abundantly in seafood, some nuts and seeds, some vegetables (particularly green leafy ones) and in grass-fed animal products. The type of omega-3 found in fish is different (and better) to that found in plants.

*Omega-6* fatty acids are found in red meat, poultry, eggs, nuts and most vegetable oils.

Both are needed for body and brain function but omega-3s are probably the most important ones for health because they suppress inflammation. In contrast to this, all but one of the omega-6s have pro-inflammation effects. So a healthy diet needs the correct balance between the two and this is around 4:1 in favour of omega-3. Unfortunately, because omega-6 is found in abundance in so many common foods *and in most vegetable oils*, the balance between the two is being distorted in the modern Western diet (see 'What is Inflammation?' in Appendix 1).

People living in Japan, thought to be one of the healthiest societies in the world, tend to eat a diet with a balance of 4:1 in favour of omega-3. This contrasts unfavourably with the balance in the typical American diet – which can be up to 1:20 in favour of omega-6!

Dr Michael Roizen (American anaesthesiologist and Professor of Medicine at the Cleveland Clinic Lerner College of Medicine) gives a graphic description of what happens when you eat too many omega-6 fats.

> [It] causes your arteries to get inflamed, causes your immune system to get inflamed, and decreases your ability to fight infections, decreases your ability to find cancer cells and get rid of them before they cause cancer, and increases inflammation and atherosclerosis in your arteries . . . Unfortunately, omega-6 fats are everywhere. We cook and bake with them; they're in packaged food, fast food, and restaurant food.[1]

**The Mediterranean diet**
It is known that an excess of omega-6 is linked to inflammation. Without a healthy balance between omega-3 and omega-6, inflammation can become chronic and lead to disease. Unfortunately, the typical Western diet over-emphasises these omega-6-rich foods whereas the traditional Mediterranean diet, one rich in olive oil, fish and vegetables, gives a healthier balance.

Some books and websites are quite alarmist about this and tell us to avoid the polyunsaturated fats found in margarines, low-fat spreads and processed vegetable oils. Google 'PUFAS' on the web and scary headlines may pop up. One of these even carries the title 'Death by Vegetable Oil'! In contrast, other books and websites are beginning to address this issue but take the line that most people have adequate amounts of omega-6 in their diet and should concentrate on eating more food with high levels of omega-3.

---

[1] http://www.cbn.com/cbnnews/healthscience/2013/April/The-Omega-Balance-Getting-Smart-about-Inflammation/

**FIBRE**

Although we all know that eating food with fibre helps keep us 'regular', there are two other things to appreciate about it:

1.  The amount of fibre in a food is one of the key factors that determines its GI value.

2.  Fibre plays an essential part in the control of cholesterol.

**What is fibre?**

Fibre is the indigestible part of plants. It is categorised as insoluble or soluble. Soluble fibre dissolves in water, insoluble fibre does not. The importance of soluble fibre in diet has only recently been fully understood through the discovery that it helps to control cholesterol levels. Cholesterol is produced by the liver. It circulates around the body in the blood and a certain amount is needed to build body cells and membranes, but too much can build up in arteries and cause heart disease.

*Insoluble fibre* is found in the skin and husks of plant food. It helps the human body to maintain a healthy digestive system. *Soluble fibre* is found in the fleshy interior of fruit and vegetables. Plants contain both types of fibre, in varying proportions. For example, plums have a thick skin covering a fleshy interior. If eaten, the skin is a source of insoluble fibre and the flesh a source of soluble fibre.

*Soluble fibre* moves through the digestive system until it reaches the large intestine (colon) where it is changed by fermentation. This slow digestion reduces the rate at which blood glucose levels rise after eating. It also reduces the amount of cholesterol produced by the liver and binds with existing cholesterol, so preventing it from being absorbed into the bloodstream. Oats, barley, legumes, linseed, chia seeds, apples and citrus fruit are all foods that contain high levels of soluble fibre.

*Insoluble fibre* is not absorbed in this way. Instead, as it works its way through the system it absorbs water and makes bowel movements easier.

## Resistant starch

Resistant starch is a carbohydrate that behaves like, and is sometimes called, the third type of dietary fibre. This is because the enzymes that turn other types of starch into glucose do not work on resistant starch. Instead of being absorbed into the bloodstream, resistant starches pass undigested into the large intestine. Foods high in resistant starch include beans, oats, sourdough bread and green bananas. Also potatoes and pasta that have been cooked then cooled. Within the bean and legume family, white beans are the best source, followed by lentils, green peas, chick-peas and kidney beans.

Food manufacturers are now on the case of resistant starch and are using it to lower the carbohydrate and blood glucose impact of their products. In their list of ingredients it may be named as 'resistant cornstarch' or 'modified cornstarch'. For example, a branded whole grain cornflour called 'Hi-Maize' containing 60 per cent resistant starch is available in the USA. Resistant starch is being added to some brands of pasta.

## Food labels: fibre

Foods labelled as 'high fibre' contain 6g or more of fibre per 100g. Adults are advised to eat 25–30g of fibre a day, of which 10g should be soluble fibre. Average adult consumption is thought to be well below this – around 14g.

The amount of fibre in a portion of food can be quite surprising. A medium-sized avocado contains 5.2g, whereas a medium-sized boiled potato contains only 1.1g. A medium dessert apple contains 3.3g. One slice of wholemeal bread contains 2.2g of fibre, one slice of white bread a mere 0.8g.

---

**FIBRE: SUMMARY**
Fibre is the indigestible part of plants.
The amount and type of fibre in a food determines how quickly it is digested.
Food containing high amounts of fibre takes longer to be digested.
Fibre also helps to control blood cholesterol levels.

---

# 3

# The Glycaemic Index

You may remember that GI stands for glycaemic index. These values were first formulated by Dr David Jenkins, a professor of nutrition at Toronto University, Canada, in 1981, and their original purpose was to give people with diabetes better control of their blood glucose levels. More recent work has been done by Professor Jennie Brand-Miller of the University of Sydney, Australia. Hundreds of foods have now been tested in laboratories and the results compiled into the present list of values.

GI values are only given to foods that contain carbohydrate and are a **measurement of the speed at which the food raises blood glucose levels**. A vast amount of technical information exists about GI values but the points to remember are that certain carbohydrates (for example, those found in large potatoes) quickly turn into blood glucose after being eaten. Foods that contain these carbohydrates have a high GI value and should be eaten sparingly.

In contrast, foods that contain more fibre take longer to be digested and have a lesser impact on blood glucose levels. These foods have a low GI value.

GI values are measured on a scale of 0–100. High GI values are 70+, medium GI values are within 56–69 and low GI values are 55 or less. GI values should always be seen as indicative. Scores frequently vary between brands and the difference of a few points between different foods will not make a significant difference.

| GI value | Category |
|----------|----------|
| 70+ | high |
| 56–69 | medium |
| 55 or less | low |

# THE AVERAGE GI OF SOME EVERYDAY FOODS

Below are the average GI values of some everyday foods:

| | |
|---|---|
| apple, raw | 38 |
| apricots, dried | 31 |
| baked beans in sauce | 48 |
| banana | 52 |
| bread, rye flour | 44 |
| bread, white baguette | 95 |
| bread, white flour | 70 |
| butter beans | 31 |
| cashew nuts, salted | 22 |
| chocolate biscuit caramel bar | 44 |
| chocolate caramel bar | 62 |
| corn flakes | 81 |
| crisps, plain, salted | 54 |
| Frosties (sugar-coated corn flakes) | 55 |
| green lentils | 30 |
| green peas | 48 |
| ice-cream | 61 |
| ice-cream, reduced fat | 37–50 |
| jelly beans | 80 |
| milk chocolate | 43 |
| milk, chocolate flavoured | 43 |
| milk, full-fat | 27 |
| milk, skimmed | 32 |
| muesli | 55 |
| new potatoes | 57 |
| orange | 42 |
| orange juice | 59 |
| parsnips | 97 |
| peanuts | 14 |
| pearl barley | 25 |
| pitta bread, white | 57 |
| plums (Canadian), raw | 24 |
| plums (Italian), raw | 53 |
| popcorn, plain | 72 |

| | |
|---|---|
| potato, mashed | 74 |
| prunes | 29 |
| raisins | 64 |
| rice, basmati | 38 |
| rice, brown boiled | 55 |
| rice, white boiled | 64 |
| Shredded Wheat | 75 |
| soya beans | 18 |
| soy milk, full-fat | 44 |
| strawberries, raw | 40 |
| strawberry jam | 51 |
| sultanas | 56 |
| sweetcorn | 54 |
| tomatoes | 38 |
| yoghurt | 36 |

GI values for foods not mentioned in the above chart can be found at www.glycemicindex.com/faqsList.php. This is a website from the University of Sydney, Australia. This website also contains questions and answers about the glycaemic index and the glycaemic load.

## THE COMPLEX CASE OF THE COOKED CARROT

The preparation of food and how it is cooked affects its GI value. Raw carrot has a low GI value of 16 but once it is diced this increases to 35. A whole carrot peeled and boiled is 33 but peel, *dice* and boil it and it increases to 49. Carrots that are boiled and *mashed* leap to a GI value of 60. These changes occur because the fibre in the carrots is being chopped up mechanically and – in the case of boiling – chemically.

But despite this, cooked carrots are still good for you, the reason being that carrots contain only a small amount of carbohydrate – the nutrient responsible for the increased level of blood glucose. So a standard portion of cooked carrot, despite its high GI, will not raise blood glucose levels by any significant degree because **only a small amount of carbohydrate will have been eaten.**

This is why some researchers prefer to use another measurement, the glycaemic load, as a predictor of blood glucose levels after eating.

## LIMITATIONS OF THE GLYCAEMIC INDEX

The glycaemic index uses a scale of 1–100 with pure glucose being the reference point at a value of 100. Values of individual food are determined by experiment. This is done by extracting 50g of the carbohydrate found in a food and giving it to human test subjects. Their blood glucose levels are then measured at specific intervals of time.

When first formulated in the 1980s the high GI values of food like white bread and potatoes came as a surprise. However, the high GI value of some foods may be misleading, as a closer look at our carrot example will demonstrate.

The average weight of a medium-sized carrot is around 78g. Of this, approximately 68g will be water, 2g fibre and only 8g will be carbohydrate. To determine the GI of carrots the testers had to extract 50g of carrot carbohydrate and, to do this, they would have needed six (and a bit) of our medium-sized carrots (6 × 8g = 48g).

But people do not eat six medium-sized carrots as a dinner portion – they are much more likely to eat just one. However, for their blood glucose to respond as predicted by the GI value of carrots, they would have to eat six carrots. If they eat just one carrot at dinner-time their blood glucose response will be much less than that predicted by the GI value. In 1997 the glycaemic load was formulated to take account of this.

# 4

# The Glycaemic Load

As we have seen, the GI value of a food does not take into consideration how much of that food is eaten. Another measure, the glycaemic load, does. This measures the effect *of a portion of food* on blood glucose levels. It is calculated using the following formula: GL = GI × carbohydrate (g) / 100.

The GL of a food is calculated for a 100g portion of that food and this leads to a high, a medium or a low GL value: high GL values are 20+; medium GL values are 11–19; low GL value are 10 or less. So, to return to our carrot example, we can now actually calculate the GL of a single carrot. We know that it contains 8g of carbohydrate and that the GI of peeled, boiled then mashed carrots is 60. A quick calculation shows that the GL of one carrot is (60 × 8) / 100 = 4.8. A GL of 4.8 is very low! We no longer need to worry about eating a cooked, mashed carrot for dinner. It will have a very limited impact on blood glucose levels.

So does this mean that a baked potato (GI 85) is okay after all? Sadly, no. As we have just seen, food with a high or medium GI *may* turn out to have a low GL. However, potatoes and many grain-based foods have high GIs *and* high GLs. **A baked potato has a very high GI (85) *and* a very high GL of 26. This tells us that one medium baked potato *will* have an immediate and significant effect on blood glucose levels.**

Many researchers prefer to use GL values but food labels tend to use GI values. One reason for this is that glycaemic loads have not been calculated for as extensive a range of foods as have GI values. However, if the GL of a food is available it is the more reliable predictor of the effect that food will have on blood glucose levels. It is worth restating that **some forms of our staple** foods, potatoes, rice and pasta, may have a medium or low GI but this can be comfortingly misleading as further enquiry reveals that they are in a higher GL category. (In a few cases this relationship works in reverse. Parsnips have a hair-raising GI score of 97 but a medium GL of 12.)

## MIXED MEALS

Meals are usually a mix of foods with different GI values. Fortunately a mix of high- and low-GI foods will result in a meal of medium GI value and this will moderate the sugar spike associated with the high-GI foods. In tests it was found that the combination of white rice (high GI) with vinegar, dairy products and beans significantly decreased the glycaemic response to the rice. This occurred whether the foods were eaten with, before, or after the rice.

## THE SECOND MEAL EFFECT

Researchers also discovered that eating a low-GI supper reduced the impact of eating high-GI breakfast cereals the next morning. This demonstrates that if a low-GI meal is eaten there is a carry-over effect to the next meal. This is because carbohydrates containing resistant starch pass through to the colon, where fermentation occurs. This has the effect of slowing down the absorption of the next meal's carbohydrates.

The best sources of resistant starch are beans and legumes. Other sources include pearl barley, bulgar wheat, sourdough bread, long-grain brown rice and green bananas. Cooking then chilling potatoes and pasta allows resistant starch crystals to form and this lowers the glycaemic response. (Recent research has shown that pasta retains this quality after reheating.)

## LIMITATIONS OF GI AND GL VALUES

Low GI values make some foods sound healthy when it is known that they are not. These are foods that are high in fat, and the reason for their low GI value is that large amounts of fat slow down the rate at which food is digested. The advice from a leading GI researcher is:

If we were to weigh the health benefits of a high GI but low-fat food (e.g. potatoes) versus one high in saturated fat but low GI (e.g. some biscuits) then we vote for the potatoes . . . the GI was never meant to be the sole determinant of what foods you choose to eat. It's essential to base your food choices on the overall nutrient content of a food . . .

(Professor Jennie Brand-Miller)

## A FURTHER WORD OF WARNING

Dr Richard K. Bernstein in his book *The Diabetes Diet* warns that some foods with a 'low' GI may cause significant blood glucose increases in people with diabetes.

---

**GI AND GL: SUMMARY**

The glycaemic index (GI) is a measure of how much a standard amount of carbohydrate (usually 50g) from a particular food will raise blood glucose level.

**High GI is 70+; Medium GI is 56–69; Low GI is 55 or below**

Foods containing a lot of fibre but a small amount of carbohydrate have a low GI.

The glycaemic load (GL) is a measure of how much the carbohydrate in a standard portion of food (usually 100g) will raise blood glucose level.

**High GL is 20+; Medium GL is 10–19; Low GL is 10 or below**

The GL is the more useful predictor than GI of the effect that certain foods will have on blood glucose levels.

Some foods have a high GI but a low GL.

Combining high and low GI foods will result in a meal with a medium GI.

Eating food high in resistant starch can reduce the glycaemic impact of a subsequent high GI meal.

Low GI does not necessarily mean low in carbohydrate. It just means that the conversion of carbohydrates to blood glucose takes longer.

Processed food with a low GI is not necessarily nutritious and is often high in fat.

Food near the upper limit of the low GI threshold may not be so good for people with diabetes.

Restaurant meals tend to be high in fat or high GI. Keep meal choices plain or vegetable based and portion size moderate.

---

# 5

# The Dietary Maze

Ok. Your fasting blood sugar test came back 'ESAJ mg/dl' which stands for 'Extra Surgery Aunt Jemima.' You said to your doctor, 'Ok, I have T2 diabetes, what can I eat?' and he said, 'Uh . . . well, uh . . . no sugar . . . and, uh . . . no potatoes or bread . . . and, uh . . . well, uh . . . you know . . . bad things and stuff like that.'

(www.digitalbirdcrap.com/diabetes)

The advice Peter received when diagnosed a few years ago was confusing. 'Eat what you like. Nothing is off limits. Just restrict how much you eat.' This was the first thing he was told during an initial visit to the doctor. The next week a dietitian told him to cut back on food like cheese, butter and sugary things but to eat as much breakfast cereal, bread and potatoes as he wanted. A leaflet given out at the doctor's surgery said that all types of bread and all breakfast cereals were fine but, at the same time, we were reading books that warned about the high GI values of food like this. We had arguments about it. I worried that Peter was eating too much bread. Peter showed me his leaflet and carried on eating the sandwiches.

The confusion persisted until I read a book by Gretchen Becker (*The First Year: Type 2 Diabetes*) in which she said that arguments about the best diet for diabetics had been going on centuries and were still going on. There is agreement that people with Type 2 diabetes should limit the amount of calories they eat and that lean meat, fish, green-leaf vegetables and other high-fibre vegetables should be a major part of their diet. The disagreements are over carbohydrates and fat, with different diets offering different advice.

## THE HIGH-CARBOHYDRATE AND HIGH-FIBRE DIET

Here fat is limited and carbohydrates that are minimally processed and contain a lot of fibre are eaten. This diet includes starchy vegetables like corn and potatoes and is the diet recommended by many nutritionists, their advice being to eat meals consisting of 20 per cent protein, 70 per cent carbohydrates and 10 per cent fat. But as it is known that the carbohydrates will turn quickly into glucose, why follow this diet? Becker explains that the diet is a trade-off. It is known that people with Type 2 diabetes are at a greater risk of heart disease. It is therefore considered that a low-fat but high-carbohydrate diet, with its attendant risk of fluctuating blood glucose levels, is preferable to the risks of a diet with a high or moderate fat content, with its attendant risk of heart disease.

## THE LOW-GI DIET

This is similar to the high-carbohydrate/high-fibre diet but more fat is allowed and carbohydrates are limited to the low-GI ones.

## EXCHANGE DIETS

These diets allow a little of everything but keep a strict count of calories and/or carbohydrates. The size and number of portions is controlled – a certain amount is allowed each day from each food group. These diets are recommended for people who do not wish to change their eating habits. Many 'diabetic' cookery books use this approach. The number of calories for a person is determined according to their weight. A small adult might be allowed 1,500 calories. Of this, 10–20 per cent would come from protein, the rest would be spread between monounsaturated fats and carbohydrates.

## THE LOW-CARBOHYDRATE DIET

For a balanced diet the GDA of carbohydrates is 300g for a man and 230g for a woman (figures correct for 2015). A low-carbohydrate diet is one in which daily intake is under 130g, and, in a very low-carb diet, daily intake is under 40g. (To put this in context, one slice of bread can contain 18g of carbohydrate, a large white potato a whopping great 58g.)

Starch and sugar are severely limited in these diets and more protein and fat is allowed. Food choices are therefore very restricted. Fruit, bread, starchy vegetables, grains – only limited amounts of these are allowed and, because of this, the diets tend to be low in calories and high in protein and fat.

So will you be hungry all the time if you follow a low-carbohydrate diet? The answer is no. Protein is more satisfying than carbohydrates so, by following a protein-based diet, you feel full (satiated) and will consequently eat less. (Try eating two boiled eggs for breakfast. You will probably not want to eat anything else for the next few hours. Do this before a day out and it will probably prevent a few visits to the snack shop.)

One high-profile writer who has Type 1 diabetes and is a believer in their effectiveness is Richard K. Bernstein (see *The Diabetes Diet*). The list of forbidden food in his diet is long and includes many everyday items. They include milk, yoghurt, fruit, all sweet or starchy vegetables including carrots, corn, onions and cooked tomatoes, wheat, oats, pasta and rice. Adhering to such a strict diet would obviously demand a fundamental change in lifestyle and eating habits.

A low-carbohydrate diet like this cannot be forced or secretly inflicted on individuals by their well-meaning wives or partners! It would need determination and will-power to follow and people may well weigh up the evidence and decide on a more moderate diet, even when this means that their diabetes cannot be controlled through diet and exercise alone. However, it is apparent from their books and blogs that the low-carb diet is the diet that many people with diabetes do choose to follow and this is reflected in the Diabetes.co.uk website, which says that an increasing amount of research is indicating that a low-carb diet is the better choice for people with diabetes.

Of course, a low-carb diet does not have to be as restrictive as Dr Bernstein's diet. A 'moderate carb' diet would be one with a daily carbohydrate intake of 130–225g a day. A diet with greater emphasis on non-starchy vegetables and less emphasis on grain-based food (bread and cereals) would be one way to approach this (with the help of a dietitian to work out the statistics).

Here are the amounts of carbohydrate in some everyday foods. More detailed information, and the amount of carbohydrate in other foods, can be found at www.glycemicindex.com/faqsList.php.

| Food | Carbohydrate |
| --- | --- |
| 1 large white potato | 58g |
| 1 sweet potato | 37g |
| 1 cup cooked white rice | 50g |
| 1 cup cooked shell pasta | 36g |
| 1 banana | 27g |
| 1 medium apple | 25g |
| 1 medium orange | 15g |
| 1 slice of bread | 18g |
| 1 cream cracker | 5.3g |
| 1 digestive biscuit | 9.4g |
| 1 Weetabix | 13g |
| 1 four-finger chocolate KitKat | 29g |
| 1 pint whole milk | 24g |

## KEY QUESTIONS

'What should I eat?' and 'How can I keep my heart healthy?' are key questions for people with Type 2 diabetes. Unfortunately, there is no doubt that, compared with non-diabetics, people who have Type 2 are at higher risk of heart disease. They have additional causes for heart disease, they may develop it at an earlier age and they may have it in more severe forms. High levels of blood cholesterol, saturated fats, unfavourable body mass index scores (see 'What is Body Mass Index?' in Appendix 1), high blood glucose levels – these may all be contributory factors. One thing is clear, however. **Just reducing calorie intake and body weight alone can be a major step towards controlling blood glucose levels and this, in itself, will help to maintain a healthy heart.**

Of course, the 'Which diet should I follow?' question still has to be answered, but at least some understanding of the issues surrounding diet should make it easier for people with Type 2 diabetes to have an informed discussion on the subject with their diabetes team. They should have access to a dietitian who can answer their questions and help them to choose the diet which best suits their medical profile and their individual circumstances. And then, whichever diet is chosen, frequent and regular testing of blood glucose levels becomes necessary. Confusion and disagreement about diet will probably persist, but people with Type 2 diabetes can be certain of two things:

1.  That diabetes is a lifelong condition and, to remain healthy, a diet of one sort or another *will* have to be followed.

2.  That reducing calorie intake alone has huge health benefits. In other words, eat less.

But, if the advice is to eat less, it makes sense to ensure that what you eat is worth eating. And, to do this, most people need to become more informed about *what* they are eating. (We did.) Here are some questions. If more people knew the answers to questions like these then perhaps different and better choices about food would be made in the supermarkets.

1.  Is there more salt in a slice of ham than a slice of white bread?

2.  Is meat from grass-fed cows different to that from grain-fed cows?

3.  Why is Greek-style yoghurt so thick and creamy and is it good for you?

4.  Is it worth paying more for eggs with added omega-3?

Discovering the answers to questions such as these has been surprising. It has led us to make further discoveries about our everyday food which, though confusing at times, has also made us more aware, and more willing to question, some of the claims made in public health announcements and in food advertising. Incidentally, the answers to the questions are:

1. Maybe
2. Yes
3. Probably
4. Maybe

If, as we hope, this leaves you thirsting for fuller answers, these can all be found in the main text of the book.

## 6

# Some Common Favourites

Traditionally the foods in this section form a major part of Western diets; unfortunately many of them are calorie rich and/or diabetic unfriendly.

## SALT

One teaspoon of salt is about 5g – just under the guideline daily amount for adults, which is 6g (6,000mg) of salt a day. Most people eat much more than this. Everyday use of the word 'salt' refers to sodium chloride or table salt. This, together with other chemicals, is now used in many food products.

Table salt is 97–99 per cent sodium chloride. It contains additives to make it free-pouring. Salt is essential for human health and development and has also become the means for preserving food and enhancing its flavour. However, too much salt is a known health risk. It can lead to high blood pressure, stroke and weight gain.

Salt is found in a wide variety of commercially produced food. Most people are aware that processed meats and smoked fish contain high levels of salt but may be surprised to learn how much is present in many brands of bread, cakes, biscuits and cereal. It might be thought that a slice of ham contains more salt than a slice of white bread. But, depending upon brand, a slice of ham can contain up to 365mg of salt, a slice of bread 400mg.

This means that one ham sandwich for lunch (taken to mean one slice of ham between two slices of white bread, no butter, no pickle, no mustard) could contribute more than a fifth of your GDA of salt. Add in the salt that may be present in your breakfast and dinner, and the amount eaten in a day is likely to exceed the recommended 6g.

The following foods will probably contain high levels of salt: packet mixes of potatoes, rice and pasta; all tinned, processed and cured meats; tinned and smoked fish; tinned soups and vegetables; ketchup, mustard and salad dressings; spreads and dips; tinned or packaged soups, gravies and sauces; pickles; olives; salty snack foods; soy and steak sauces; food containing monosodium glutamate (MSG).

## POTATOES AND ROOT VEGETABLES
### Why you may need to cut back on potatoes
Potatoes are an important part of many people's main meal of the day, but a serving of mashed potato will raise blood glucose levels quickly. This is because potatoes are very high in the type of starch that gets digested very quickly.

The GI value of potatoes varies according to variety and type of cooking. The highest GI value is in potatoes that are freshly cooked, mashed or baked. Pre-cooking and reheating or eating cold cooked potato (for example, in potato salad) has been shown to reduce the glycaemic response by as much as a third.

White potatoes and waxy potatoes contain lesser amounts of carbohydrate than red-skinned varieties. Small new potatoes are a better choice because, the younger they are when picked, the lower the carbohydrate content (and this is true of all fruit and all vegetables).

|  | Average GI | GL |
|---|---|---|
| Baked potato | 85 (high) | 28 (high) |
| Chips | 75 (high) | 30 (high) |
| Mashed potato | 74 (high) | 15 (medium) |
| Sweet potato | 61 (medium) | 17 (medium) |
| New potatoes | 57 (medium) | 12 (medium) |
| Boiled old potatoes, cold | 56 (medium) | no known data |
| Potato crisps | 54 (medium) | no known data |

The average GI values of potatoes cooked in different ways

These are average figures. There are single studies that give chips a much lower GI value of 51 and mashed potato a higher value of 85. The variations may be due to factors like variety of potato or thickness of the chips. Whatever the reason, it is a reminder that GI values are indicative only.

### Should people with Type 2 diabetes give up potatoes?

Well, a large daily portion of mashed potato is probably not a good idea. But rather than giving up potatoes, the types of potato and the way they are eaten can be altered. Instead of cooking big starchy potatoes, small potatoes can be cooked in their skins, cooled and then reheated. And mashed potato does not have to totally disappear – it can become a mixed mash. A medium potato can be left unpeeled, cut into chunks and boiled while a similar quantity of broccoli or cauliflower is steamed on top. The two can then be mashed together. Generous amounts of spinach or kale can be included in a potato mash, or equal amounts of potato and beans mashed together – these are all ways of reducing the glycaemic response to big starchy potatoes. And don't forget bubble and squeak – a medium potato cooked with a generous number of sprouts, mashed and then fried and served with a poached egg on top is a quick supper. As always, **a moderate portion rather than a mountain of mash is key**.

Cooking potatoes like this may seem fiddly and time-consuming but, in theory, it reduces the glycaemic response that mashed potato alone will elicit. Rightly or wrongly (no research evidence here), it makes us feel able to eat small portions of mashed potato without feeling guilty or anxious. Unfortunately, the same cannot be said of baked potatoes or chips – there is no way they can be turned into a low- or even medium-GL food.

### But remember – the skins are good for you

Potato skins contain a lot of fibre. They also contain high levels of potassium and vitamin C as well as other beneficial substances. It is known that potassium is linked to a lower risk of heart disease and stroke, but only if the potassium comes from natural food. As supplements taken in pill-form do not confer this benefit it makes sense to cook potatoes in their skins whenever possible. Roast potatoes are the only ones that really need to be peeled.

### Potato crisps
These have a medium GI but are likely to contain a lot of salt – between 0.5–1g of salt for every small (30g) packet.

### Sweet potatoes
These are not members of the potato family. They have a medium GI value but are considered nutritious because they contain high amounts of beta-carotene – the substance that makes carrots orange. Sweet potatoes take the place of ordinary potatoes in many low-GI recipes.

### Parsnips
Parsnips have a GI of 97, almost as high as glucose. But, as parsnips have a medium GL of 12, a small portion of parsnip should not have the same undesirable effect on blood glucose that a small portion of mashed potato has.

## THE PIZZA EFFECT
Many people have reported that eating pizza causes their blood glucose levels to climb completely out of control and there is now scientific confirmation that pizza does indeed raise blood glucose levels higher, and for a longer period, than other high-GI foods. The exact reason for this is almost certainly connected to the highly refined white flour base of a pizza.

## SO CAN I EAT RICE?
GI values of most rice varieties range between medium and high (with the exception of 'converted' rice, which is low). White rice is from the same plant as brown rice but has had its husk and bran removed by milling. The inner part is very starchy. Brown rice has had only the outer husk removed so contains more fibre (as well as vitamins and minerals). Long-grain brown rice is a source of resistant starch and has a lower GI than white rice.

Basmati rice (like converted rice) has a higher amylose (a resistant starch) content than other types of rice so should be low or medium GI but this is not always borne out when researched on the web.

A healthy portion of uncooked rice is around 50g per person.

*Doongara* long-grain rice is a recent addition to the rice market. White or brown SunRice Low-GI Rice, available online, has a GI of 54 – just within the low range. It is a new Australian variety produced specifically for its low GI, similar to basmati but with a lower starch content.

*'Converted'* rice has been parboiled in a special patented manner. The grains are pressure steamed, then dried, and this forces all of the nutrients from the husk of the rice into the starchy bit. The husk falls off. The rice granules that are left are highly nutritious and, because they contain very high amounts of resistant starch, have the exceptionally low GI value of 38.

Converted or parboiled rice can be difficult to find. It is not available in UK shops but can be bought online. Uncle Ben's Original Converted Enriched Parboiled Long-Grain Rice, available from Amazon, is £27.69 for a 5kg bag. It cooks quickly, is less sticky than other rice and is quite chewy and filling.

It is difficult to make direct comparisons between the GI levels of various types of rice because published values for them vary so much, but a very rough average is given below.

| Type of rice | GI | GL |
| --- | --- | --- |
| Long-grain white rice, boiled | 64 (medium) | 23 (high) |
| Pre-cooked basmati rice in pouch, white, reheated in microwave | 57 (medium) | 23 (high) |
| Brown rice, boiled | 55 (low) | 18 (medium) |
| Basmati rice | 52 (low) | no known data |
| Doongara long-grain rice | 54 (low) | no known data |
| Converted rice | 38 (low) | no known data |

## BREAD: CAN YOU SEE THE SEEDS?

Look up any of the hundreds of websites about bread and most will tell you that bread made with refined white flour has a very high GI, will cause a rapid spike in blood glucose levels, contains unwelcome additives and contributes very little in the way of nutrients.

Bread, and how much of it to eat, is a contentious subject for people with diabetes. There may be advice to fill up on carbohydrates, including bread. Other information sources may recommend a much more moderate carbohydrate intake.

Bread made with wholemeal flour, with added seeds, with sourdough, and rye and barley breads, granary and multigrain breads all have a lower GI value than plain white bread. A dense, dark pumpernickel loaf, made with rye flour, has a particularly low GI.

The list of ingredients on the label of a supermarket loaf rather than its name will provide the information needed to make an informed choice. The term 'wholemeal' by itself is meaningless. The bread may have more nutrients than ordinary white bread but the flour is still highly refined. Bread with a lower GI will have a high percentage of whole grain or wholemeal flour and a high fibre content. The entire grain of wheat, including fibre, is only found in whole grain (granary) bread.

### The GI and GL of some types of bread

The published data on GI values for bread varies between brands. As an example, the GI for whole grain bread varies between 53 and 70, depending upon the manufacturer. The values in the chart below are therefore just a guide.

This chart might suggest that some types of bread, products with a low GL, can be eaten without worry by people with Type 2 diabetes. But, before deciding to do this, it is worth noting that many people who have the condition choose to drastically reduce the amount of bread they eat, even bread made with whole or coarse grains. They report that all grains seem to elevate their glucose levels disproportionately to the amount of bread they have eaten.

| Type of bread | GI | GL |
|---|---|---|
| Baguette, white | 95 (high) | 15 (high) |
| White bread, wheat | 70 (high) | 10 (low) |
| Hamburger bun | 61 (medium) | 9 (low) |
| 100 per cent whole grain | 59 (medium) | 7 (low) |
| Pitta bread, white | 57 (medium) | 10 (low) |
| Corn tortilla | 52 (low) | 12 (medium) |
| Pumpernickel (rye) | 53 (low) | 5 (low) |
| Wheat tortilla | 30 (low) | 8 (low) |

## Switching from white

Although it may be beneficial to cut out bread altogether, and some people are able to do this, for the others it is good advice to choose wholegrain bread and to eat it in moderation, two to four slices a day only. Some brands to try are Co-op Wholemeal Seeded Batch Loaf (8.5g fibre per 100g), Vogel Wholemeal and Oat with Fibre (9.7g fibre per 100g), and Hovis Seed Sensations (12.4g fibre per 100g).

Bread is often eaten in the form of sandwiches and, if eaten with low-GI foods, the glycaemic response to the bread can be reduced. An alternative to a sandwich is a wholemeal tortilla. The ratio of healthy filling to carbohydrate can be much greater in a wrap than it is in a bread sandwich.

For the people who love sandwiches and cannot do without them, try to reduce the impact of the bread by turning it into a mixed meal. Make open sandwiches on rye, sourdough or pumpernickel bread and pile on the topping. Or make a many-layered sandwich with a thin layer of spread, a protein layer (cheese, peanut butter, hummus, meat etc.) and a vegetable layer (slices of onion, tomato, beetroot, cucumber, gherkin etc.).

**Bread machines**

It may take some time and experimenting to find the recipe that best suits your machine but once done a bread machine can really change shopping habits. It takes just five minutes to throw in the ingredients for a small loaf. Then, with one touch of a button, the kneading, putting aside to rise etc. is all done for you. Homemade bread tends to be denser. It fills you up more and this helps to prevent return visits to the bread bin.

## SWEET BISCUITS

Probably never a healthy choice but the better ones are plain sweet biscuits with a low or medium GI. Traditionally these have been Rich Tea and digestives. But be aware that digestive biscuits contain quite a lot of salt. (Reduced-fat versions of these biscuits can be found.) Newer varieties with a lower GI, called 'breakfast biscuits', are now on the market. BelVita (Kraft Foods) produce biscuits which are made with whole grain flour and contain more fibre. Weetabix produce 'on the go' biscuits, made with wheat and oats. Nairn's produce mixed berries oat biscuits which are wheat free.

## IS BREAKFAST CEREAL OKAY?

Maybe, but most breakfast cereals are high GI. The packets are designed to make the contents look natural, wholesome and healthy but a quick check of the label will show that most of them are made from highly refined grain and are packed with sugar. Cornflakes, Rice Krispies, Shredded Wheat, Weetabix and puffed wheat all have GI values that are high or very high.

Alpen (no added sugar), Special K, Sultana Bran and All-Bran all have low GIs but remember Dr Bernstein's concern that some 'low' GI foods significantly raise blood glucose levels in people with diabetes. Milk in any form is low GI so this will reduce the impact of a bowl of cereal. The GI of porridge made with oats can vary between 40 (low) and 60 (medium), depending upon the extent to which the oats have been processed. The GI of instant porridge can vary between 65 (medium) and 85 (high).

The best breakfast cereals are those with oats as their main ingredient, and sugar a long way down the list of ingredients. The addition of nuts and seeds will lower the GI but dried fruit, particularly dates, may increase it. Careful reading of labels makes it possible to find cereals with sugar below 15g per 100g and fibre above 7g per 100g.

*Muesli* is a breakfast cereal based on uncooked oats with added fruit, nuts and seeds. It originated back in the 1900s when Dr Bircher-Benner, a Swiss doctor, 'invented' it for his hospital patients. Presented with a bowl of Dr B-B's muesli now, people would probably pull a face. It consisted of a tablespoon of rolled oats soaked in water, a tablespoon of lemon juice, a tablespoon of condensed milk and one large sour apple, grated and mixed in.

Commercially produced muesli is often high in sugar but it is easy to make your own and you then have a healthier breakfast. *Granola* (high GI) is basically muesli with added rice or maple syrup.

## PASTA: BETTER *AL DENTE* OR COLD, THEN REHEATED
Pasta is mostly carbohydrate. Italian-style dried pasta is made from a hard type of wheat called durum, which digests quite slowly. This is why pasta is sometimes said to have a low GI. The GI of pasta actually depends partly on its shape. The thicker the pasta the lower its GI. Also relevant is the way it is cooked – longer cooked (therefore softer) pasta has a higher GI than pasta that is *al dente* (i.e. food that is still firm to the bite – not totally soft or soggy). Most pastas are in the GI range of 40 to the low 60s but are likely to have a higher GL than might be expected. Cooked, chilled then reheated pasta has been found to have a significantly lower glycaemic response.

| Pasta type and cooking method | GI | GL of 180g |
|---|---|---|
| Couscous | 65 (medium) | no known data |
| White spaghetti, boiled 20 mins | 58 (medium) | 26 (high) |
| Lasagne sheets, white | 55 (low) | no known data |
| White spaghetti, boiled 11 mins | 46 (low) | 22 (high) |
| Wholemeal spaghetti, boiled | 42 (low) | 17 (medium) |
| Fettuccini, boiled | 32 (low) | 15 (medium) |

## Keep an eye on portion size

The carbohydrates contained in pasta trickle into the bloodstream for hours after they are eaten. Because of this they may not cause the pronounced blood sugar spike that a baked potato or white bread produces. However, the carbohydrates in pasta still need to be metabolised and, if they are not burnt off through exercise, they are likely to turn into fat. For this reason, whatever its GI, dietitians still recommend that the consumption of pasta should be limited. The dry weight of a portion should be about 40g which gives a serving of half a cup of cooked pasta. This would have the comfortingly low GL of 7 (an average for pasta as a whole). But most people eat portions far larger than this and, if your serving of pasta is more like two cupfuls (the average restaurant-sized portion), then you cannot fall back on the comforting thought that you are eating a low-GL meal.

Fresh pasta is made with regular flour. This is the type of pasta usually served in Italian restaurants. It digests much quicker than dried pasta and will produce the sugar spike associated with white refined flour.

Some pasta manufacturers are now trying to reduce the GI and increase the nutritional value of their product. Pasta made from spelt flour is available from some health food shops. Another possibility is to add protein. Pasta 'plus' products claim to be lower in carbohydrates because they include flour and/or fibre made from sources other than wheat. It is rumoured that pasta made from green banana flour will become available sometime.

*Couscous* has a high GI value of 65. It is a type of pasta, made from semolina – a flour which is produced from durum wheat during the pasta-making process.

### To cook *al dente*
The length of time pasta is cooked has a significant impact on blood glucose. Just one minute past *al dente* will make a noticeable difference and the softer the pasta the higher its impact. To cook *al dente*, test the pasta a minute *before* the minimum cooking time on the label has passed.

### Reheat your pasta
It has been known for some time that the carbohydrate in pasta, when cold, turns into a resistant starch, which takes a long time to break down into blood glucose. (A similar process occurs with cooked, then cooled, potato.) This means that cold pasta has a lower GI than hot, freshly cooked pasta. The even better news is that reheated pasta retains this quality and has an even lower GI than cold pasta. Recent research found that the blood glucose levels of people who eat reheated pasta was up to 50 per cent lower than people who eat pasta freshly cooked.

### To sum up
If you have time, cook your pasta *al dente*, leave to cool, then reheat. Add protein and lots of vegetables to further reduce impact on blood glucose levels.

### NOODLES
Noodles made from rice are high GI. Wheat and buckwheat noodles are medium GI. 'Zero Noodles' are a Japanese brand which are 96 per cent water. A 100g serving contains just five calories. Similar products can be purchased cheaper at Asian stores under the name of shiritake or konjac noodles.

### BUTTER
Butter contains cholesterol (a substance found only in animal products) and high levels of saturated fat (around 50 per cent).

Commercially produced butter also contains around 20 per cent of monounsaturated fat.

In most people the cholesterol they eat in food does not adversely affect their blood cholesterol levels. But, as we have just seen, butter also contains high amounts of saturated fat and this does continue to be problematic.

There are now conflicting opinions about whether the statistical connection between saturated fat and heart disease is a causal one. Mary G. Enig, the researcher who gave early warning about the danger of trans fat, held the view that certain saturated fats, such as those found in butter and coconut oil, are both necessary and beneficial.

To keep things in perspective, in the UK butter and other fat-spreads make up about an eighth of a person's daily fat intake. Meat (processed meat in particular) and cheese are a far bigger source of fat, particularly saturated fat.

## Types of butter
'Whipped' butter (butter with added air) is lighter and less dense than block butter and contains up to half the calories.

'Light' butter (made with added air and water to replace the butterfat) contains half the fat and calories of block butter.

Butter blended with vegetable oil (usually olive or canola oil) has lower levels of saturated fat and cholesterol. An example is Lurpak Spreadable.

## Buttermilk
Originally buttermilk was the whey left after the butterfat had been removed from milk. Commercial buttermilk is now made by adding bacteria to low-fat milk and leaving it to ferment at a low temperature. It has a slightly sour taste – similar to yoghurt – and has a similarly low GI. This is sold as cultured buttermilk and often contains salt. Buttermilk has many uses, for example

in baking, salad dressings and marinades. It makes particularly good scones.

## MARGARINE

The original butter substitute, created in 1869 in France, was made of beef tallow and skimmed milk. Margarines today are made from refined vegetable oils or are a combination of vegetable oil and milk fat. 'Spreads' have added water. By the 1960s margarine had become a major part of our diet and butter was getting a very bad press. But some people now argue that, by substituting spreads or margarine for butter, we are replacing good nutritious food with food that may be harmful. Butter, they say, is a natural product with a wonderful taste, margarine a synthetic factory mix of oils and additives that tries, unsuccessfully, to taste like butter.

Margarines contain high levels of omega-6 and other poly- and monounsaturated fats. Like all fats they are high in calories. In the past hard margarines contained trans fat – formed when hydrogen was added to vegetable oil to turn it into a solid. It is now recognised that this was a dangerous practice but traces of trans fat may still exist in some products. Since 2012 many of the big firms operating in the UK have pledged to eliminate all traces of trans fat from their products. Margarine manufacturers are now promoting soft tub margarines which overall contain less fat but more of the monounsaturated and omega-3 type.

Some margarines and spreads have plant stanols and sterols added to them. These are substances that occur naturally, but in very small amounts, in some grains, fruit, seeds and nuts and they are known to have powerful cholesterol-lowering properties. Some food manufacturers are now adding them to products. Two examples are Flora pro-activ (a spread) and a range of spreads and yoghurts from Benecol.

## CHEESE

Milk from animals is fermented to make cheese. Milk itself is made up of proteins, carbohydrates and fats, whereas cheese is mostly made up of fat and protein. This is because the carbohydrates get used up during fermentation and, as there is little or no carbohydrate left after fermentation, the end product (cheese) does not have a GI value.

It may come as a surprise that Cheddar cheese contains significantly more fat than Brie or Camembert cheese. Goat's cheese is lower in fat and has fewer calories than cow's milk cheese. Nearly all varieties contain high levels of saturated fat and some cheeses contain high levels of salt. For example, 1oz/25g of typical Cheddar cheese contains 176mg of salt whereas 1oz/25g of reduced-fat Cheddar can contain over twice as much. Presumably, extra salt has been added to replace the flavour that has been lost by reducing its fat content.

It's not all bad news for cheese-lovers. Cheese is a good source of protein and calcium. The protein can curb hunger and the calcium keeps teeth and bones strong. Cheese also contributes other nutrients when it is eaten as part of a controlled and

| Type of cheese | per cent fat content |
|---|---|
| Reduced-fat cottage cheese | 0.5 |
| Cottage cheese | 4 |
| Ricotta | 12 |
| Reduced-fat Cheddar | 15 |
| Feta | 16 |
| Mozzarella | 18 |
| Camembert | 22 |
| Bri | 22 |
| Edam | 25 |
| Parmesan | 30 |
| Cheddar | 35 |
| Cream cheese | 37 |
| Blue cheese | 41 |
| Mascarpone | 47 |

The fat content of different types of cheese

balanced diet. It should not be used as the prime ingredient too often as it is high in calories but small amounts of the stronger cheeses especially can often be used to give flavour.

## Low or reduced-fat cheeses

Low-fat cheeses are made from milk which has been skimmed to remove the cream, and as it is the cream which carries much of the taste of a full-fat cheese they will not taste as rich as their full-fat counterparts.

# FLOUR AND DERIVATIVES

## Flour

Flour is created when a dry grain is milled or pounded into a powdery substance. It is often made from wheat but can be made from any grain. Flours vary according to how much of the original grain is used in the milling process. It may include the bran (the outer layer), the endosperm (the bulk of the grain) and the germ (the embryonic shoot of a new plant). The endosperm is the starchy bulk of the grain and is the only part that is used in simple white flour. Bran adds texture, colour and fibre. The germ is high in nutrients, vitamins and fibre. Gluten is found in wheat flour and gives the characteristic elasticity of bread dough.

Refined white flour is bad news for people with Type 2 diabetes. The husk of the wheat grain, which contains fibre, vitamins and minerals, has been removed and the remaining part (almost entirely endosperm) has a dramatic effect on blood glucose.

Brown flour has had 85 per cent of its bran and germ removed. Wholemeal flour uses all of the grain. Stone-ground is wholemeal flour ground between two stones. Wheat, barley and rye flours contain gluten – the protein which binds dough during cooking and causes it to rise. Wheat contains particularly high levels of gluten.

## Some alternative flours

The gluten-free flours include *cornflour*, *buckwheat*, *soy and rice flour* and *polenta*. Some people believe that a gluten-free diet can help to reduce the symptoms of Type 2 diabetes. (People who suffer from coeliac disease are allergic to gluten and have to use gluten-free products. It has been estimated that one person in a hundred has coeliac disease and one person in six has gluten intolerance.)

*Spelt flour* is a gluten-containing member of the wheat family. It comes just within the low GI range, and contains slightly fewer calories and slightly more protein than wheat flour. It can be used as a substitute for white flour in bread, biscuits, cakes and pastry – sift two teaspoons of baking powder into 150g of spelt flour to make it 'self-raising'.

## Nut flour
*Ground almonds* sometimes feature in low-GI recipes for cakes and puddings. But ground almonds also contain quite a lot of omega-6 – it is estimated that 100g of almonds gives 12g of omega-6.

*Coconut flour* may be a healthier option. It is made from finely ground coconut meat with most of the moisture removed. It has low levels of omega-6, is gluten free, contains high levels of protein, is very high in fibre and has a low GI. The saturated fat content is 20 per cent. The flour is very dry. It actually behaves rather like a sponge, and recipes using it need more liquid than other flours. Research shows that replacing just some wheat flour with coconut flour when baking lowers the glycaemic response to the cooked product.

*Soy flour* is made from ground roasted soybeans. It is full fat, low fat or defatted. Some writers describe soy as a superfood with almost miraculous health benefits, including very low GI values, while other writers suggest it is responsible for a range of health problems.

## Pastry
Commercial pastry is usually made with refined white flour, is high in fat and has the very high GI value of 84. Sweet pastry has added sugar. So visits to the pie shop really are rather dangerous.

Low-GI recipe books sometimes include savouries or desserts made with filo pastry. This is because just two or three sheets of filo lightly sprayed with olive oil is thought to be a healthier alternative to shortcrust or flaky pastry. Homemade pastry that includes some low-GI flour should produce pastry with a lower glycaemic response but there is no published data about this.

| Flour type | Average GI |
|---|---|
| Rice flour | 95 |
| Refined white | 85 |
| Polenta | 70 |
| Whole meal | 66 |
| Spelt | 54 |
| Rye | 45 |

Average GI Values of Some Types of Flour

## RED MEAT

Red meat is a rich source of protein. It provides a lot of iron and all essential amino acids. However, red meat also contains high levels of saturated fat and cholesterol and moderate levels of omega-6. The advice now is to eat meat sparingly, to buy lean cuts and to cook it using low-fat methods.

'But our grandparents used to eat red meat every day and lived to a good old age.' This is the argument frequently made by those who enjoy their daily quota of meat and veg. The trouble is that our grandparents did much more exercise than us and cows used to eat grass! This is not such a flip response as it might appear because **the meat most of us eat now is not the same as the meat our grandparents would eat.** Vegetarians aside, unless we buy organic (which is expensive), most of us eat meat that is produced from grain-fed animals. But this presents problems. By changing traditional farming methods to one based on grain-fed animals we are, in effect, fattening *ourselves* up on grain. Grain-fed meat contains more fat, more omega-6 and less omega-3 than grass-fed meat.

Different types and cuts of meat contain different amounts of omega-6, and pork and chicken contain more than beef. But, put in context, it is still a relatively small amount compared to the level in processed vegetable oil.

Whether red meat is good or bad is a contentious subject but, as the general advice now is to eat less, perhaps it would be to everyone's benefit (including the animals') if we bought less but better-quality meat. Yes, meat from grass-fed livestock is more expensive than the grain-fed alternative, but it is leaner and it is more nutritious.

**Grass-fed meat**
The marketing-label 'grass-fed' refers to animals that, except for their mothers' milk, have been fed solely on grass or forage for all of their life. It has been estimated that a 6oz/150g steak from a grass-fed animal contains 100 less calories than a similar-sized steak from a grain-fed animal. It also contains higher levels of omega-3 fatty acids and lower levels of omega-6. In addition, grass-fed meat contains up to four times more vitamin E (an antioxidant), and meat and milk from grass-fed cattle are the richest-known source of a beneficial fat called conjugated linoleic acid (CLA). There is emerging evidence that CLA reduces the risk of cancer in humans.

**Antibiotics**
There are other advantages. Animals raised organically are not given antibiotics, bovine growth hormones or other drugs. Nor were they forced to eat their own kind (giving cattle the ground-up remains of cow carcasses in the 1980s was found to be one of the causes of mad cow disease). Today, poultry, pigs and cattle kept in mass-production 'farms' are fed low levels of antibiotics daily – this is to promote growth, to compensate for their poor living conditions and to prevent sickness, which would spread rapidly. To what extent do these hormones, antibiotics and whatever else is fed to intensively farmed animals enter the food chain? Answers are hard to come by:

'The meat industry doesn't publicize its use of antibiotics, so accurate information on the amount of antibiotics given to food animals is hard to come by' ('Antibiotic Debate Overview': http://www.pbs.org/wgbh/pages/frontline/shows/meat/safe/overview .html).

There are calls for the practice of routinely giving animals antibiotics to cease (it is already outlawed in some European countries) and, in 2013 the Health Minister Anna Soubry called on farmers in the UK to stop the practice, but no legislation has been passed.

### Processed meats
Processed meats contain additives, in particular salt, nitrates and nitrites, whereas fresh meat is naturally low in salt – typically it has 100mg per serving or less. Processed meats vary in the amount of salt they contain but it can be up to four times this level. Some examples are:

| Product | Mg of salt – the GDA for an adult is 600mg a day |
|---------|--------------------------------------------------|
| One pork sausage | 178 |
| One hotdog | 250 |
| One slice of regular ham | 365 |
| One slice of corned beef | 476 |

*Is processed meat particularly bad for us?*
Yes, and the research points to fat content, salt and sodium nitrite. This is a chemical used to preserve the colour of meat. Fresh meat, when cooked, goes grey, so why does processed meat and bacon remain looking so pink and fresh? Answer – it has probably been treated with sodium nitrite. This chemical is used to inhibit the growth of micro-organisms and, as one of the really bad ones causes botulism, this is clearly necessary. But, unfortunately, sodium nitrite interacts with the digestive acid found in our stomachs to make nitrosamines, and these are chemicals that may cause cancer. Evidence of this indirect link between sodium nitrite and cancer is not yet conclusive but

consumers should be aware.

## Sausages

Sausages have a bad reputation, fully deserved in the case of low-quality ones which are full of fat, salt and other additives, and contain little meat. However, better-quality sausages often use cuts of meat that might otherwise be wasted and can have a high meat content of 80–90 per cent. All sausages, good or bad, contain preservatives, salt, flavourings and other additives but a couple of meat-rich sausages, served with lentils or beans and lots of vegetables, still make a nutritious meal for loyal sausage-lovers.

## SUGAR

Most people know that we are eating too much sugar. We eat naturally occurring sugar in fruit and milk and our bodies are designed to cope with this. But the modern diet also includes high levels of 'free sugars' and these are not so good for us.

### 'Free sugars'

The sugars added to food by manufacturers, and by us in the kitchen, are called 'free sugars'. These include syrup and honey and they do not contrast favourably with the natural sugars found in fruit, vegetables and milk. This is because foods containing natural sugars also contain micronutrients – vitamins, minerals and fibre – which contribute to a healthy diet. Free sugars contribute calories only and therefore dietitians recommend that their intake be limited.

## SUGAR SUBSTITUTES

Sugar substitutes are substances that replicate the taste of sugar but with fewer calories. They can be natural or synthetic.

Ordinary table sugar is called sucrose and is made from sugar-cane or sugar-beet. The body converts it into glucose. Sucrose has a GI value of 60–65. *Fructose* is the most common sugar found in fruits, vegetables, honey and other foods, including corn. It has the much lower GI value of 19.

## NATURAL SWEETENERS

These include fructose, honey, rice syrup, maple syrup, stevia and Palmyra Jaggery. Agave nectar is also marketed as a natural sweetener.

### Fructose or fruit sugar

Packets of this can be found in health stores. It is granular and tastes like sugar but is metabolised very differently by the body. Fructose has a low GI because it goes straight to the liver, where it is metabolised.

### High fructose corn syrup (HFCS)

This is a product that is derived from corn starch. It is very cheap to produce and is now a major source of added sugar in the modern Western diet. Consumption of too much fructose is now associated with (among other things) **metabolic syndrome**. This is a pre-Type 2 diabetic condition which is characterised by too much fat in and around the abdomen, 'sticky' blood and raised blood pressure.

Under normal conditions, consumption of the fructose that occurs naturally in products like fruit is not a health issue. But the excessive consumption that now occurs is different and some researchers believe that the rise in obesity and the increasing number of people with diabetes in Western society is directly linked to the prevalence of HFCS in so many products. High fructose corn syrup is now found on the labels of a vast range of foods and it has been estimated that the average American consumes sixty pounds (27.2 kilograms) of it every year. Studies have indicated that 25 per cent of the American population have metabolic syndrome.

### Agave nectar

Agave nectar is a syrup made from the large bulbous root of a plant grown in Mexico. It is up to one and a half times sweeter than table sugar. Because the process which converts the starch of the agave root to syrup is a chemical one, some people question whether agave nectar should be called a natural sweetener. The sugar which it produces is similar to fructose and has a correspondingly low GI.

## Honey

The GI value of honey is 55. It contains a high amount (around 55 per cent) of fructose.

## Jaggery

This is any unrefined sugar made from sugar-cane or palm tree sap and is widely used as a sweetener in the Indian subcontinent. The most nutritious is *Palmyra Jaggery*, made from Palmyra (a type of palm). This contains a lot of sucrose but only a small amount of fructose. It is intensely sweet but is low GI (40). There are other benefits. It contains a number of nutrients, particularly vitamin B, calcium and iron. It is sold as a syrup or in powder form and is expensive (at the time of writing, £7.99 for 250g from Conscious Foods, marketed as SugaVida). Check the label and buy only unadulterated Palmyra Jaggery – some manufacturers add sugar-cane jaggery (molasses), as this is much cheaper.

## Maple syrup

The GI value of maple syrup is 54. Content-wise it is nearly 70 per cent sucrose.

## Rice syrup

The sugar in rice syrup is glucose and is therefore likely to have a high GI value (there is no published data for it yet). The syrup is highly processed and high in calories and carbohydrate. Organic brown rice syrup is increasingly being used as an alternative to high fructose corn syrup in manufactured foods. There is a question mark over its use – some researchers suggest that harmful levels of arsenic can build up in the processing procedure. Many cereals, cereal bars and infant formulas contain rice products.

## Stevia

Stevia comes from the leaves of a plant that is native to Paraguay and has been used in cooking in that country for hundreds of years. The sweetener that comes from its leaves is almost 300 times sweeter than table sugar. Because of its concentrated sweetness stevia is usually blended with a bulking agent so that it can be measured and used as a substitute for table sugar. It has a metallic after-taste. Stevia has a zero GI value and contains zero calories. However, the bulking agent may not have a particularly low GI or GL value.

Sweeteners containing stevia are sold in UK supermarkets. Truvia was developed by Cargill and Coca-Cola. Tate & Lyle have a product called Light at Heart. This contains stevia with table sugar as its bulking agent, resulting in a GI value that is similar to sugar (sucrose) but less of it needs to be used to achieve the same level of sweetness.

Some stevia products contain very little stevia. These products have erythritol as their main ingredient and this is a sugar alcohol manufactured from genetically engineered corn. Whether to use them or not depends upon your attitude to sugar alcohols as they can cause stomach upsets in some people. Pure stevia powder can be purchased but people who try it often complain of a bitter after-taste.

### Whey Low
This is made from lactose (milk sugar), fructose (fruit sugar) and sucrose (table sugar). It is only available in the USA and Canada. It is a 'natural' product that tastes like sugar because it *is* sugar! Mainly fructose, Whey Low is low in calories, has a low GI and can be used in cooking as a straight substitute for sugar. It is expensive. A 2lb packet of Whey Low Granular currently costs $12.99.

## SUGAR ALCOHOLS
Neither sugar nor alcohol, these are types of carbohydrate with a chemical structure that resembles both sugar and alcohol, hence their misleading name. Sorbitol, maltitol and xylitol are all common examples.

Although sugar alcohols occur naturally in plants, they are mostly manufactured from sugars and starches. Sugar alcohols are sweet but do not behave like sugar. Because of this, food containing sugar alcohols can be labelled 'sugar-free'; the alcohols are frequently used in the manufacture of chewing gum, sweets, cakes, biscuits and soft drinks. Sugar alcohols have fewer calories than sucrose and have a lower GI. After eating, sugar alcohols turn to glucose quite slowly and do not cause sugar spikes. But they do still contain carbohydrates so are not a blank cheque as they still have some effect on blood glucose levels. In this respect they are dissimilar to artificial sweeteners, which are calorie free and have no effect on blood glucose.

Sugar alcohols do not cause tooth decay and xylitol actually prevents bacterial growth in the mouth. This is why they are often used in toothpastes and mouthwashes. In other respects the different types of sugar alcohols act on the body in different ways. Most of them are less sweet than sugar so more is needed to get the same degree of sweetness. Over-consumption of sugar alcohols can lead to diarrhoea, bloating and weight gain.

### Sorbitol
A natural substance found in some fruits, including prunes. Once widely used as a sugar alternative, it is now known that over-consumption of sorbitol is unwise for people with diabetes. This is because sorbitol is not metabolised in the body, so if a lot is eaten in the form of food additives it can build up to dangerous levels in the blood. It can then result in serious diabetic consequences – nerve damage, problems with vision and blood-vessel damage.

### Xylitol
A natural substance found in fibrous vegetables, fruit, corn-cobs and some hardwood trees. Commercial xylitol is made mostly from corn-cobs. It is considered safe but amounts higher than 30g per day can cause stomach discomfort in some people. It is widely used in brands of toothpaste and chewing gum.

The sugar substitute Total Sweet is a brand of xylitol. It is advertised as having a GI of 7 and 40 per cent fewer calories than sugar (see www.totalsweet.co.uk). Total Sweet tastes like sugar – there is no after-taste, and it performs well in baking. It is expensive, at £10–£12 per kilogram at the time of writing.

**Warning: xylitol is deadly to dogs. If they eat products containing xylitol, dogs can become weak, uncoordinated and suffer seizures, with liver and brain damage occurring within twenty-four hours.**

### Erythritol
This is created from fermented glucose but is not metabolised by the body. Instead it goes almost unchanged through the digestive system (about 90 per cent of ingested erythritol is excreted unchanged in urine). For this reason it is thought to be less likely to cause digestive upsets than other sugar alcohols although some people may be more sensitive to it than others. Erythritol is used as the bulking agent for several stevia products. An example is Truvia, which has no glycaemic effect and is popular as it can be used as a straight sugar substitute. (Truvia does have a slight after-taste which may be discernible if used in tea or coffee but it is not so apparent in cooked products.)

## SYNTHETIC SWEETENERS
Artificial non-calorie sweeteners are high-intensity sweeteners that have many times the sweetness of sucrose. Their use means that people with diabetes can enjoy a more varied diet and still keep control of their sugar intake. These sweeteners are now found in many commercially produced food products, particularly those labelled as 'lite' or 'sugar-free'.

Synthetic sweeteners vary in the degree to which they are absorbed by the body. Commercially available artificial sweeteners have all been extensively tested and passed as safe but, despite this, many people still think they pose a health risk. They are made from chemicals that would not have been encountered in pre-industrialised society, and some scientists question whether the human body can properly tolerate them. Research suggests that some people are more tolerant of them than others and that some synthetic products can trigger conditions like migraine.

Examples of synthetic sweeteners are sucralose and aspartame.

## Sucralose

A chlorinated sugar compound (this means it is made from sugar), sucralose is a widely used artificial sweetener. NewSweet and Splenda are examples. It is 400–800 times sweeter than table sugar and therefore requires a bulking agent. It has a clean taste and is minimally metabolised by the body (around 85 per cent passes directly through the system into bowel movements, and most of the remainder is eliminated in the urine). The safety aspect of sucralose has been extensively investigated and most studies indicate a lack of risk. However, some people experience adverse effects at very high levels of intake.

Splenda contains only a small amount of sucralose. It uses dextrose and maltodextrin (both glucose derivatives with a very high GI) as a bulking agent. This could make it unsuitable for people with diabetes.

## Aspartame

So far it has been possible to give readers some understandable idea of what sugar substitutes are made from. This is not so easy with aspartame, unless you are a chemist. Wikipedia tells us that it is a methyl ester of the aspartic acid phenylalanine dipeptide. It is 200 times sweeter than table sugar and is said to be the one that comes closest to the taste of sugar among all approved artificial sweeteners. Aspartame has had more complaints than any other food additive. Products containing it have been linked with numerous side-effects – especially migraine, but also nausea, stomach irritation, rashes and depression. However, science and speculation relating to aspartame can be difficult to tease apart, and most research suggests that it is safe. AminoSweet is aspartame under a different name.

## CONFUSED ABOUT SUGAR AND SUGAR ALTERNATIVES?

You will not be alone. The supermarket shelves are now laden with choice. It is obviously best to try to reduce the urge to eat something sweet, but this is easier for some people than others. Attitudes about non-natural sugar substitutes tend to polarise. Some people are vehemently anti, others take a more pragmatic approach and trust the food authorities that label them as safe (though it should be remembered that newer sugar substitutes have not been around long enough for research into their long-term effects.

Before deciding which ones to use, the product label should be checked for ingredients, accompanied by a quick look on the web to get fuller information. And don't just look on the product's own website – find independent reviews. To help in the choice, opposite is a list of ingredients that occur (not all at the same time) in some popular sweeteners:

## FRUIT JUICE

This is the last of our 'common favourites'. Pure fruit juice is much higher in sugar than fresh fruit and contains little or no fibre. Juice drinks (as opposed to pure fruit juice) are worse as they usually contain added sugar, often in the form of high fructose corn syrup.

The glycaemic load of 8oz/200ml of unsweetened orange juice is 9. This is just within the low range. As 8oz/200ml fills a medium-sized glass this means that a drink must be restricted to one glass to keep within this low range.

The advice to people with diabetes is to check the label on fruit juices for their sugar content, to limit consumption of juice and/or to drink it diluted with water. Tomato or vegetable juices have fewer carbohydrates and fewer calories. Fruit juice freshly squeezed at home is a healthy alternative to commercial juice. Citrus fruits all have low GI values compared to other fruits and, if the pulp is included in the drink, can also be a source of soluble fibre.

| Substance | What is it? | Where is it? |
|---|---|---|
| Aspartame | A synthetic sweetener | Canderel<br>Half Spoon<br>NutraSweet<br>Tesco Granulated Sweetener |
| Erythritol | A sugar alcohol | Truvia |
| Maltodextrin | A bulking agent obtained from corn starch | Canderel<br>Splenda<br>Stevia Sweet (Tesco)<br>Tesco Granulated Sweeteners |
| Steviol glycosides | A chemical found in stevia leaves | Light at Heart<br>Truvia |
| Sucralose | A synthetic sweetener | NewSweet<br>Splenda<br>Tesco Low Calorie Granulated Sweetener |
| Xylitol | A sugar alcohol | TotalSweet<br>Life is Sweet |

## CONCLUSIONS

Some of our favourite foods, often eaten daily and unthinkingly, benefit from a closer, slightly critical look. These foods are often high in rapidly digested starch – the type that turns quickly into glucose. Other things to consider are the additives (including sugar) that are often added to food, the type of fat that a food contains and also the style of cooking.

---

### SOME COMMON FAVOURITES: SUMMARY

Watch the salt content of food: it's probably higher than you think.

Small potatoes are the best. Eat them cold or reheated.

Pizza will give you a spectacular sugar spike.

Choose basmati rice if you are a supermarket shopper; doongara or converted rice if you are willing to go online.

White bread has a GL higher than sugar! The denser the bread the lower its GL.

Oat-based breakfast cereals are the best. Check the label for sugar.

Cook your pasta *al dente*, chill then reheat it.

Butter or margarine? Butter is high in saturated fat, margarine is high in unsaturated fat, both poly and mono. Some margarines have added sterols and stanols – cholesterol-lowering substances.

Do you know the fat content of your favourite type of cheese?

Refined white flour has the very high GI of 85. Mix in some wholemeal, spelt, coconut or soy flour to reduce it.

Eat less but better red meat. Consider buying organic.

Sugar substitutes can be natural, sugar alcohols or synthetic. There is now a vast range to choose from, although the best advice is to tame the urge to eat something sweet.

Look out for 'free sugars'. Avoid food that contains them.

Commercial fruit juices usually contain high levels of free sugar. Consider diluting them or juicing citrus fruits at home.

---

# 7

## Good Foods (With a Few Provisos)

### FISH

Fish is highly nutritious as it provides many of the nutrients found in meat without the disadvantages of meat. White fish is low in fat and high in protein. Oily fish (for example, salmon, mackerel, trout, sardines and pilchards) are higher in fat than white fish, a high proportion of this being omega-3 – the type of polyunsaturated fat known to protect against heart disease. Fish also contains the one 'good' omega-6 fat known to have an anti-inflammatory effect. People are advised to eat up to 12oz/300g (two to three portions) a week of a variety of fish and shellfish – one of these an oily fish.

Tinned fish contains as much protein as fresh, although tuna may lose its omega-3 oils in the canning process. Prawns and other shellfish contain omega-3 but not as much as oily fish. Smoked salmon has all the benefits of fresh salmon but contains a lot of added salt. Kippers count as an oily fish but are also high in salt.

### Mercury levels in fish

Mercury is released into the air from industrial pollution. When it gets into water it is turned into methyl-mercury and fish accumulate this as they feed. Nearly all fish and shellfish contain traces of methyl-mercury, but some species more than others, depending upon their position in the food chain and their size. Shark, swordfish, king mackerel and tilefish all contain high levels of mercury. Fresh tuna contains more mercury than tinned. Fish and shellfish that contain low levels of mercury include salmon, prawn, crab and lobster and canned light tuna (albacore or 'white' tuna contains higher levels).

People who regularly eat types of fish high in mercury can

accumulate it in their bloodstream. Methyl-mercury is removed from the body naturally but it can take up to a year for levels to drop. Pregnant women and young children are advised to limit their consumption of fish known to contain mercury.

## VEGETABLES

At last! Things to eat without having to worry about anything. No saturated fat, no cholesterol, no wondering if those annoying omegas are in balance. Instead, six good reasons to eat vegetables:

1. They are high in fibre. Fibre binds with cholesterol in the blood and removes it from the body; fibre also lowers the glycaemic response and promotes good digestion.

2. They are high in potassium and other health-giving minerals and vitamins. This gives protection against some forms of cancer.

3. They contain antioxidants (see 'What are Antioxidants?' in Appendix 1). These help to reduce ageing and tissue damage.

4. They contain high levels of omega-3. These are needed to restore a good balance with the omega-6 contained in other food.

5. They provide a non-calorific feeling of fullness. This helps keep the weight off.

6. They taste good. True, some are a bit boring but the more imaginative cookbooks usually find original ways to spice up the more bland-tasting ones.

Reading this you might think 'Hmm. Perhaps it would be safer to live on vegetables.' It has been tried. It is called The Gorilla Diet and you need to eat over 9kg of vegetables a day. Just think how much time it would take to collect and then eat 9kg of raw mixed veg, and then the time that would be spent in the toilet!

And you would still be lacking in protein, fat, and certain nutrients and vitamins (real gorillas get these from termites and caterpillars), all of which are necessary for body and brain health. So no, you can't live on vegetables alone, although most people would probably benefit from eating far more vegetables than they do.

The best vegetables are the dark green leafy ones or the brightly coloured ones. These are high in antioxidants and flavonoids. So large helpings of spinach, carrots, lettuce, cabbage, broccoli, cauliflower, tomatoes, peppers and peas are all good for you. Large helpings of starchy vegetables, such as potatoes, are not. So choose vegetables that grow above the ground, not those that grow below (except carrots).

Research done at Leicester University (2012) suggests that eating the green leafy vegetables like broccoli, spinach and kale reduces the risk of Type 2 diabetes. The high levels of magnesium in these vegetables is thought to help regulate blood glucose levels.

Vegetables are best eaten unpeeled and raw or lightly steamed. Tinned and pickled vegetables may contain a lot of salt, and too much of this is known to narrow blood vessels and increase blood pressure. However, studies indicate that vinegar slows down the digestion of carbohydrates, which makes pickled vegetables a good choice. Beetroot, for example, contains a lot of sugar. It has a high GI (64) but a low GL of 4 and the GL of beetroot in vinegar would lower it further.

The peel of vegetables should be eaten for its fibre content. The amount of fibre in a vegetable depends on which bit of it is eaten and how it is prepared. One cup of cooked peas contains 8.8g of fibre, one cup of cooked sweetcorn contains 4.2g. This is significant because fibre, particularly soluble fibre, lowers blood cholesterol levels and reduces the GI of food.

# Is it worth buying organic?

Research at Newcastle University has shown that organic crops contain up to 60 per cent more key antioxidants than non-organic crops. In addition, they contain lower levels of toxic heavy metals. These findings were for organic fruit, organic vegetables and organic cereals and for food made from them.[2]

## The five best

An organisation called Food Day gave vegetables scores based on their nutritional content, and the vegetable with a score far, far higher than any other vegetable was kale. The next best (but with much lower scores) were spinach, carrots, purple sprouting broccoli and then broccoli heads.[3] Cooks suggest that dinosaur kale (Latin name *Lacinato kale*) is the best. Long used in Italian cooking, dinosaur kale has dark blue-green leaves which are more delicate and slightly sweeter than curly kale.

## MUSHROOMS

These are not vegetables. Mushrooms are fungi, densely packed with beneficial minerals and with greater antioxidant benefits than most vegetables, even the brightly coloured ones. A quirky ability that mushrooms have is to absorb sunlight and turn it into vitamin D. So let your mushrooms sunbathe on a sunny windowsill for an hour or two before cooking.

## AVOCADOS

Because these carry the seed of the tree, they are considered a fruit. Avocados contain a lot of monounsaturated fat and are high in calories but are packed with health-giving minerals and vitamins. One medium-sized avocado contains 30g of fat and 15g of fibre. It has a GI of 15 (low). The ratio of omega-6 to omega-3 is high (15:1); the actual amount of omega-6 in an average-sized avocado is about 1.6g.

---

[2] http://www.ncl.ac.uk/press.office/press.release/item/new-study-finds-significant-differences-between-organic-and-non-organic-food, July 2014.

[3] www.buzzfeed.com/deenashanker/find-out-which-vegetables-are-the-best-for-you.

## PICKLE ALERT

Despite being vegetable based, some varieties of chutney and pickle contain a lot of sugar. Sweet brown pickles can contain up to 26 per cent of sugar. A piccalilli-type pickle contains less — around 13 per cent of sugar.

## VINEGAR

Several research studies indicate that vinegar can reduce the glycaemic response to high-GI food, possibly by as much as 50 per cent.[4] The researchers suggest that two tablespoons of vinegar before a high-carbohydrate meal will help to reduce the sugar spike that follows.

The beneficial substance in vinegar is acetic acid and this will be found in any type of vinegar although apple cider vinegar is most likely to be promoted for its health benefits as well as its taste. Unpasteurised apple vinegar also contains healthy probiotics. Apple cider vinegar can be infused with fruit (raspberries are popular) to make fruit-flavoured vinegars.

Taking doses of straight vinegar is not an appealing prospect but vinegar can be used for salad dressings, or added to salads or pickles (but pickles must be low-sugar ones to gain this benefit).

## SALAD CREAM OR MAYONNAISE?

Salad cream usually contains less fat and has vinegar as its first ingredient, whereas mayonnaise has vegetable oil as its first ingredient. We have just seen that vinegar can lower the glycaemic response; we know that vegetable oils contain a high amount of omega-6 — something that most people could probably do without. Neither can be called healthy, but salad cream may be the better choice. (Low-fat mayonnaise contains around the same amount of fat as salad cream.)

---

[4] http://care.diabetesjournals.org/content/27/1/281.full. See article 'Vinegar Improves Insulin Sensitivity to a High-Carbohydrate Meal in Subjects With Insulin resistance or Type 2 Diabetes'.

## LEMON JUICE

Some people suggest that lemon juice has a similar effect on blood sugar levels as vinegar. For this reason diabetes websites may recommend a regular drink of water mixed with 1oz/25ml of lemon juice before a meal. Bottled lemon juice is said to work as well as fresh.

## FRUIT

Fruit for pudding can be okay if the portion is not large. An example of the portion size recommended by dietitians is two fresh apricots.

Different types of fruit contain differing proportions of fructose and sucrose, and the amount of sucrose in a fruit increases as it ripens. Fruit provides many beneficial nutrients, including flavonoids (see 'What are Flavonoids?' in Appendix 1), vitamins and fibre, but because of their sugar content people with diabetes are advised to eat no more than two or three portions over the course of a day. Fruit eaten on an empty stomach is likely to cause a sugar spike. Fruit that is very high in sugar (e.g. over-ripe bananas) should be eaten sparingly.

The high GI of some fruits can be misleading, as the chart opposite shows.

### Apples and citrus

These contain a high amount of soluble fibre – beneficial because it slows down digestion, reduces the rate at which blood sugar levels rise after eating, and works to eliminate cholesterol from the body. One medium-sized apple contributes 20 per cent of a person's daily fibre requirement, which is the equivalent of a bowl of bran cereal. As a bonus, apples are also full of cancer-beating antioxidants. But some apples are much sweeter than others – varieties like Pink Lady contain more sugar and may not have such a low GI. *One medium apple or two satsumas = one portion.*

| Fruit | Average GI | GL |
|---|---|---|
| Watermelon | 72 (high) | 4 (low) |
| Cantaloupe melon | 65 (medium) | 4 (low) |
| Pineapple | 59 (medium) | 8 (low) |
| Black grapes | 59 (medium) | 11 (medium) |
| Apricots | 57 (medium) | 5 (low) |
| Banana (ripe) | 52 (low) | 13 (medium) |
| Mango | 51 (low) | 9 (low) |
| Kiwi fruit | 47 (low) | 6 (low) |
| Orange | 42 (low) | 5 (low) |
| Peach | 42 (low) | 5 (low) |
| Strawberries | 40 (low) | 2 (low) |
| Blueberries and raspberries | 40 (low) | 5 (low) |
| Apple | 38 (low) | 6 (low) |
| Pear | 38 (low) | 4 (low) |
| Grapefruit | 25 (low) | 3 (low) |
| Cherries | 22 (low) | 3 (low) |

### Berries
All the berries (black, blue and red) contain high amounts of flavonoids. Their low GI depends upon being eaten with no added sugar. *Ten to twelve berries = one portion.*

### Bananas
Bananas are high in iron, potassium and fibre and are known to be a mood-lifter. Size matters – small bananas contain significantly less carbohydrate.

### Grapes
Grapes, sometimes called sugar-bombs, have a high sugar content and are generally labelled as bad for diabetics. However, grapes – especially red and black ones – also contain compounds that have health benefits. Overall, grapes can be considered to have a medium GI so long as only a few are eaten. *Eight to ten grapes = one portion.*

### Grapefruit
Grapefruit are either yellow or pink skinned. They have a low GI value of 25 and provide a big hit of vitamin C. The pink varieties

contain a much higher concentration of vitamins and minerals, some of which have antioxidant properties. Pink grapefruits get their colour from lycopene – a substance that has the ability to fight the compounds in the body that cause cell damage. In fact, pink grapefruit are so full of beneficial things that they are sometimes called a superfood.

However, **grapefruit and prescription drugs may not mix**. The list of drugs that grapefruit interact with in a negative way is long and advice should always be taken from a doctor. A commonly prescribed class of drug that interacts with grapefruit is statins. People taking statins must avoid grapefruit in any form as one of the compounds in the fruit will prevent the absorption of the drug, resulting in a dangerous accumulation of the drug in the body.

### Dried fruit

Prunes and apricots are the best. Dried fruits are generally about 50 per cent fructose. Some are low GI but most have a higher GL. The dehydration process that removes water from fruit makes it shrink and concentrates the sugar, so dried fruit, even if it has a low GL, is high on calories. Raisins, with their high GL, are not so good for a snack as is sometimes thought – dried apricots are a better choice. Cranberries have a GI ranging between 20 and 60, according to variety. (This is because sugar is usually added to cranberries before the dehydration process.)

| Fruit (brand not specified) | Average GI | GL |
| --- | --- | --- |
| Currants | 64 (medium) | 9 (low) |
| Dates | 62 (medium) | 41 (high) |
| Figs | 61 (medium) | 19 (medium) |
| Sultanas | 56 (medium) | 25 (high) |
| Raisins | 54 (low) | 28 (high) |
| Dried peaches | 35 (low) | no figure |
| Dried apricots | 30 (low) | 9 (low) |
| Prunes | 29 (low) | 10 (low) |
| Dried apple | 29 (low) | no figure |

Prunes, with their very low GL, would probably not be a popular choice as a snack but they add flavour and sweetness to Moroccan type meat dishes and, chopped, can replace some of the raisins and sultanas in a mixed fruit cake.

## EGGS

Egg yolk contains cholesterol and it used to be thought that the consumption of too many eggs increased the risk of heart disease. This advice was relaxed when evidence became available that dietary cholesterol is not directly related to blood cholesterol levels.

An egg is mostly water. An average size-6 egg weighs 53g and consists of: protein 12.8 per cent; fat 10.1 per cent, of which saturated is 3.1 per cent; carbohydrate 0.3 per cent; water 76.8 per cent.

It is now thought that eggs are good for you. They are a complete protein as well as being full of essential vitamins and minerals. Eating an egg can control hunger and blood glucose levels as it will satisfy the appetite for a longer period.

When deciding which eggs to eat, an important point to consider is where they have comes from. Free-range eggs from chickens fed a natural diet are more nutritious than battery eggs as they contain up to twenty times more omega-3. Eggs also contain omega-6 – quite a lot. Research into a supermarket egg discovered that the ratio of omega-3 to omega-6 (ideally something like 4:1) is more like 1:19. So, if possible choose organic free-range eggs – the eggs are more nutritious and the chickens live a more humane life.

## MILK

Milk, part of our diet for centuries, is a complete food with high levels of minerals, protein, vitamins etc. Full-fat milk does not contain a huge amount of fat; only 3–5 per cent of it is fat, while the fat content of semi-skimmed is even lower – 1–2 per cent. Cow's milk is about 87 per cent water.

All dairy products contain slow-to-digest carbohydrates in the form of sugars. The carbohydrate in milk is known as lactose. After consumption, lactose is broken down in the small intestine to form glucose. Milk also contains protein and fat, which slows digestion. The fat in full-fat milk will slow the process even further, which is why the GI of milk is in the low range, depending on fat content. Lactose intolerance – a digestive difficulty where people are unable to digest the sugars found in milk – makes milk consumption difficult for some people, who may, however, be able to eat cheese or yoghurt.

## YOGHURT

Plain yoghurt has a GL of 11, Greek yoghurt a lower GL of 5. The difference between the two is that Greek yoghurt is strained to remove the liquid whey from the source milk and it is this process that makes it thick and creamy. It takes more milk to produce Greek yoghurt – for this reason it contains more protein than plain yoghurt and is more expensive to produce.

| Nutrient per 1 tablespoon | Greek yoghurt | Low fat plain yoghurt |
|---|---|---|
| Protein | 2.6g | 1.9g |
| Carbohydrate | 2.2g | 3g |
| Fat | 4.6g | 0.4g |
| Kilocalories | 60 | 22 |
| Calcium | 57mg | 65mg |

A recent Cambridge University study (February 2014) suggests that eating one small carton of low-fat yoghurt five times a week can significantly reduce the risk of developing Type 2 diabetes. Fermented dairy products seem to give some degree of protection because they contain beneficial bacteria and a special form of vitamin K. Research has shown that food containing live cultures (probiotic) helps to control blood glucose.

## OATS

These have a higher nutritional value than nearly any other grain. They contain protein and vitamins and also provide soluble fibre that helps to lower cholesterol levels. It is a shame then that flour made from oats cannot be used to make bread. This is because oat flour does not contain gluten so will not hold together or rise in the baking process. Traditionally, oats were eaten as a cooked gruel or porridge.

Oats are marketed under different names, according to the extent to which they have been processed. And, of course, the more processed they are, the greater their loss of nutrients.

*Groats* are whole oat kernels that have been de-husked and toasted. They contain nearly the whole nutritional value of the grain.

*Steel-cut oats or Irish oats* are groats which have been cut into two or three pieces.

*Scottish oatmeal* is groats that have been cut into many more pieces.

*Rolled (jumbo) oats* are made by steaming and flattening the groats with a roller.

*Instant or quick oats* are highly refined and may be packaged with salt and sugar.

The GI of porridge made with oats varies between 40 and 60, depending upon the extent to which the oats have been processed. The GI of instant porridge can vary between 65 (medium) to 85 (high).

### Eating more oats
Oats can be substituted for some of the flour in bread, cakes, biscuits and crumbles. Oat-based breakfast cereals can be made at home or purchased in supermarkets. Oatcakes can be used for snacks in place of bread. Oat-based drinks to replace milk can be found online and from health stores. Oatly Oat drink is made from oats and water with added calcium and vitamins. Oatly Organic Creamy Oat is an alternative to cream.

# BEANS, PULSES AND GRAINS

Supermarkets now sell the seeds, beans and lentils that used to be found only in health food shops. They come in a wonderful range of colours, shapes and sizes. Typically they contain protein, high levels of slowly digested and resistant starch and fibre, and are low in fat. Most of them are low GI. They contain both omega-3 and omega-6 fatty acids but the ratio can be an unbalanced one, with high levels of omega-6 and little omega-3.

Beans, lentils and split peas all belong to the legume family. A legume is any plant that has seed pods that split along both sides when ripe.

Beans from packets must be soaked before cooking. This hydrates them and removes toxins. Tinned beans should be rinsed to wash off the salt used in the canning process. The label on tinned beans should be checked, as some have a very high sodium (salt) content.

## Lentils

Lentils are the dried seeds of an Indian plant. They do not need soaking before cooking so are quicker to use than beans. Lentils come in a variety of colours. All are highly nutritious but green and brown lentils contain twice as much fibre and more health-enhancing minerals than red ones. Red lentils break down more quickly into a purée.

## Split peas

Split peas (green or yellow) are the dried seeds of an Asian plant that naturally divide when peeled. Green split peas are used to make green pea and ham or bacon soup. Yellow split peas are used to make daal. Like other legumes, split peas contain a lot of protein and fibre.

## Chick-peas

Chick-peas, one of the earliest known cultivated vegetables, come from a Middle Eastern plant with one pod containing two to three peas. Dried chick-peas have a long cooking time – up to two hours. This can be reduced by pre-soaking but, again, they need a long time – up to twenty-four hours.

## Quinoa
Quinoa (pronounced keen-wah) is the seed of a South American plant and, unlike other seeds, is a complete protein, containing all the essential amino acids. When cooked, it is crunchy and slightly nutty. Quinoa quadruples in volume after cooking and can be used as a substitute for rice or potatoes. It is also sold as a flour and has the low GI value of 52.

## Flaxseed or linseed
High in omega-3, antioxidants and other important nutrients, flaxseed can be added to bread dough, muffin mixes etc. but needs to be ground up before use, otherwise it is difficult to digest.

## Chia
Chia is a member of the mint family and is grown for its seeds. It is native to Mexico and Guatemala. The word chia means oily and chia seeds are rich in omega-3. They also provide protein, fibre, antioxidants, soluble and insoluble fibre. Chia seeds have no flavour and can be added to muesli or bread mixes. Health food shops usually stock small packets.

## Pearl barley
Pearl barley is barley with the outer layer of inedible husks removed, then polished to remove its bran layer. It has the very low GI value of 19 and is high in fibre. Barley that has not had its bran removed is called hulled, pot or Scotch barley; it is chewier than pearl barley and takes longer to cook.

## Bulgar wheat
Bulgar wheat has a GI value of 48. It is usually made from durum wheat and is sold parboiled and dried, with most of its bran retained. It has a high nutritional value.

### Cracked wheat
Cracked wheat is crushed wheat grain that has not been parboiled.

### Freekeh
This is wheat, harvested when young and then roasted. It contains fibre and resistant starch. Whole grain freekeh has a GI of 43, cracked freekeh a GI of 55.

### Buckwheat
Buckwheat is a member of the sorrel and rhubarb family. Commercially grown buckwheat comes largely from China. The large triangular seed of the plant is processed to make noodles and flour. Buckwheat flour is gluten free, high in fibre and contains many health-giving minerals. It has a strong, slightly bitter taste and a GI value of 54.

### A word of warning
Don't get too excited by the high omega-3 content of some seeds. **The type of omega-3 fatty acids derived from plants is not as beneficial to humans as the omega-3s that are obtained from oily fish.** This is because the type found in seeds and plants contains less of the really good stuff which is essential for healthy brain function, skin and eyes. To get technical about this, the two really crucial omega-3s are DHA and EPA and these are found primarily in certain types of fish. Another type of omega-3, named ALA, is found in plants. Humans can convert ALA into DHA and EPA – *but not very efficiently*. The best way to get good levels of DHA and EPA is from eating oily fish.

Chickens *are* able to convert ALA into the good stuff. So chickens that are fed a special diet of flaxseed and other plant material can produce eggs that have exceptionally high levels of DHA and EPA. These eggs are marketed as omega-3 eggs with the label DHA + EPA on their packaging.

## PRODUCTS WITH ADDED OMEGA-3

Some foods are being advertised as having added omega-3. But the type being added to food is often the ALA type and this is not nearly as beneficial as the DHA and EPA type. The advice from independent websites is that, unless it is DHA and EPA that is being added, it is not worth paying extra.

## SOY

Soy is a complete protein and the properties of the bean have attracted much scientific interest. Soy protein is thought to reduce the risk of heart disease, cancer, osteoporosis and other diseases and for this reason is sometimes called a superfood. The beans are low in saturate fats, high in protein and fibre, a source of calcium, iron, magnesium, several vitamin B compounds, antioxidants and a natural compound that actually lowers levels of bad cholesterol and increases levels of good cholesterol. Soy beans have the lowest GI value of any food. However, soy beans in their natural state also contain a large number of dangerous toxins, the main one being phytate (found in all varieties of raw bean). Phytates interfere with the digestion and absorption of certain nutrients from food. Soy beans also contain high levels of omega-6.

Strong opinions exist about soy. It is regarded as a wonder food by some, but as others regard it as a dangerous hormone-disrupting evil, it is a controversial food. Soy has been used in Asia for centuries but the use of highly processed soy in so many products today is new. Soy can be in cakes, biscuits, breads, sausages, ready meals, margarine . . . the list goes on to such an extent that processed soy is actually quite difficult to avoid! It has been estimated that soy exists in 60 per cent of all processed food.

There have been many health scares about soy-derived food but extensive research has concluded that it is safe to eat because processing and fermentation removes the dangerous substances in the bean. However, some soy products may be better than others – highly processed soy is likely to have had many of its nutrients stripped away.

Foods containing soy include soy milk, cream, yoghurt and butter; soy flour, soy nuts and tofu. Soy beans can be used as a substitute for other types of bean. Soy flour can be used to thicken gravy and sauces. A tablespoon or two of soy flour can be substituted in muffin or cake recipes and soy milk, cream and yoghurt can be used as a substitute for their dairy equivalents. This includes using them in cooking (they have a higher GI than their dairy equivalents). Soy nuts are made from soy beans that have been soaked in water, then compressed and baked. They look like small brown nuts and can be used to replace nuts in recipes.

### Using soy as a dairy substitute
Different brands have different tastes. If soy milk is being used instead of dairy milk it is important to make sure the brand chosen has added calcium.

### Tofu
Tofu is made by separating soy milk into curds and whey. The curds are then pressed into a solid. Tofu ranges in density from firm to soft. It is flavourless and takes on the flavour of whatever is cooked with it.

### Soy sauce
Soy sauce is a condiment produced by fermenting soy with certain bacterial moulds and salt. There are many varieties, all with distinctive characteristics. Miso is soy fermented with fungus and salt. A study has shown that Chinese dark soy sauce contains ten times the quantity of antioxidants found in red wine. It may also contain anti-allergy properties.

## CHOCOLATE
It may be welcome news that a small amount of dark chocolate is probably good for you. Really dark chocolate (cocoa solid 70 per cent +) contains high levels of flavanols which help to reduce blood pressure and increase levels of good cholesterol. However, restraint is still necessary – 6g of dark chocolate per day

(equivalent to one small square) is thought to give the benefit of chocolate without raising other health risks.

## COFFEE
Rather confusingly, studies indicate that coffee is both good and bad. Some research suggests that caffeine makes it more difficult to keep blood glucose levels stable, other research suggests that people who drink a lot of coffee have a lower risk of diabetes than other people.

One explanation for this is that caffeine is not the agent responsible for any beneficial effect — some other component of coffee is. It is now established that caffeine can disrupt the control of blood glucose levels whereas decaffeinated coffee appears to help keep levels under control.

## CINNAMON
Cinnamon is widely used in traditional medicine for a variety of ailments and it is now thought that compounds in the spice may help the body to use insulin more efficiently and lower blood glucose levels. Cinnamon may also have anti-inflammatory properties and may have the ability to lower levels of 'bad' cholesterol.[5]

Powdered cinnamon is usually a mix of cinnamon and cassia (a member of the same botanical family but with a stronger taste. Cassia also contains coumarin — a compound with blood-thinning properties. Consumption of large amounts of cassia cinnamon should be avoided.) Cinnamon is often used in baking. It is also a common ingredient in savoury dishes from North Africa and the Middle East. True cinnamon comes from Sri Lanka and is more expensive than cinnamon mixed with cassia.

[5] http://care.diabetesjournals.org/content/26/12/3215.full. article 'Cinnamon Improves Glucose and Lipids of People With Type 2 Diabetes'.

It is possible to buy cinnamon supplements from health stores but always discuss with a health professional before deciding to try them.

## TURMERIC

Widely used in India as an ingredient in curries, there is now a suggestion that turmeric can cancel the possible negative effect of eating high levels of rice and flour breads. Normally these would raise blood glucose levels quite dramatically but researchers have discovered that curcumin, the active ingredient in turmeric, may help to control high blood glucose, high cholesterol and inflammation. Discuss with a health professional before deciding to try it.[6]

## WHITE MULBERRY LEAF

Some of the chemicals found in white mulberry leaves are similar to those found in medicine used to control diabetes, and powder or tablets made from it is being marketed as a means of reducing blood sugar spikes when taken before meals. It is a common ingredient of Far Eastern medicine, where it is used for a range of other conditions. Because it is a relatively new supplement no long-range studies have been done. Discuss with a health professional before deciding to try it.[7]

## CONCLUSION

This chapter suggests that fish, especially oily fish, vegetables, some grains and pulses, and moderate amounts of fruit are all good choices that can be eaten without too much worry. Dairy products, if they agree with you, and eggs can also be seen as natural wholesome foods that have been part of our diet for centuries although milk intolerance is a problem for a growing

[6] http://www.di.uq.edu.au/turmeric-and-type-2-diabetes. See article 'Turmeric could be the link to treating type 2 diabetes'.

[7] http://care.diabetesjournals.org/content/30/5/1272.full. See article 'Influence of Mulberry Leaf Extract on the Blood Glucose and Breath Hydrogen Response to Ingestion of 75g Sucrose by Type 2 Diabetic and Control Subjects'.

number of people. Coffee and chocolate may offer certain health benefits. Supplements using cinnamon, turmeric and white mulberry leaf may also offer health benefits, but always check with a health professional before trying them.

---

**GOOD FOODS (WITH A FEW PROVISOS): SUMMARY**

Oily fish gives the benefit of the better omega-3 fatty acids.

Vegetables are full of fibre, flavonols and antioxidants. They are good for you – especially the brightly coloured ones.

Recent research has shown that fruit, vegetables and cereals grown organically contain higher levels of antioxidants and lower levels of toxic heavy metals.

A small dose of vinegar reduces the glycaemic response.

Fruit is full of fibre, flavonols, antioxidants and sugar. People with Type 2 diabetes should eat no more than two to three portions a day, spread out over the day.

Dried fruits tend to have a high GL. Prunes and apricots have lower GLs than raisins and sultanas.

Free-range eggs contain more omega-3 and less omega-6 than battery eggs.

Full-fat milk is not a high-fat food. All types of milk are low GI.

Eating plain no-sugar yoghurt regularly may help to prevent the onset of Type 2 diabetes.

Oats are the most nutritious of all grains.

Beans, pulses and grains contain high amounts of fibre. Most are low GI.

The omega-3 found in nuts and seeds is not as beneficial as the omega-3 found in oily fish.

Soy is sometimes called a superfood because of its range of health benefits. Not all writers agree.

Eating a small square of plain chocolate each day may be good for you.

Decaffeinated coffee may help to control blood glucose levels.

Certain spices may help to control blood glucose levels.

---

# 8

# Foods Which Might Be Okay

## NUTS

It is easy to become confused about nuts. Google the question 'Are nuts good for you?' and many websites say yes. Nuts have a high fat content (typically around 80 per cent) but it is the 'good' type that can raise levels of 'good' and lower levels of 'bad' cholesterol in the blood. But, Google the question 'Do nuts contain too much omega-6?' and the answer will also be yes. Nuts contain little or no omega-3 but moderate to high levels of omega-6, depending upon variety. The ratio between the two omegas is therefore a poor one – a *very* poor one in some cases. So a diet containing large amounts of nuts could result in an unbalanced diet that causes inflammation. A balanced diet should contain one part of omega-6 to four parts of omega-3, written as 1:4. Here are some ratios. In all these examples the first figure refers to omega-6 content:

| | |
|---|---|
| Walnuts | 4:1 |
| Macadamias | 6:1 |
| Pecans | 20:1 |
| Pistachios | 37:1 |
| Hazelnuts | 88:1 |
| Cashews | 117:1 |
| Pine nuts | 300:1 |
| Brazil nuts | 1000:1 |
| Almonds | 1800:1 |

These figures are quite startling. Does this mean that almonds contain a massive amount of omega-6 and we should not eat them? This is where it becomes confusing. A quarter-cup of almonds (in other words, a snack-sized portion) contains the relatively modest amount of 4.4g of omega-6. Compare this to a similar-sized snack of walnuts. These have a healthier ratio of 4:1 omega-6 to omega-3 but our walnut snack actually contains 9.5g of omega-6.

## The amount of omega-6 in a snack-sized portion (quarter cup)

| | |
|---|---|
| Pine nuts | 11.6g |
| Walnuts | 9.5g |
| Brazil nuts | 7.2g |
| Pecans | 5.8g |
| Almonds | 4.4g |
| Pistachios | 4.1g |
| Hazelnuts | 2.7g |
| Cashews | 2.6g |
| Macadamias | 0.5g |

These figures seem to suggest that almonds are a healthier snack than walnuts. But are they? Research is now suggesting that a daily handful of walnuts gives some protection against Alzheimer's disease. Does this mean that we have to choose which disease it is more prudent to guard against?

Having explained all this, it may now be best to forget it, or at least not get too worked up about it. Our remote ancestors would have regarded nuts as a treat. Nuts would have been seasonal, difficult to find and then fiddly to get at. But unshelled nuts are now readily available and it has become too easy to eat too many. If we regularly binge on nuts we are likely to put on weight (a cupful of mixed nuts contains around 600 calories) and consume too much omega-6. But if we consider nuts a treat, to be eaten a few at a time, then we can benefit from the many nutritious things that they also contain without worrying too much about the negatives. Nuts contain minerals, vitamin E and antioxidants, each type of nut containing a different mix of nutrients.

Some writers are concerned about the way food is becoming over-analysed and broken down into parts. This, they say, over-simplifies food and fails to give the total story. Natural food is a bundle of natural goodness which should be looked at as a whole. Nuts are a good example. Yes, they may be high in omega-6. But they also contain many other nutrients, including antioxidants and, if a whole nut is eaten, these antioxidants may give the body protection against the inflammatory effect of the omega-6.

## Nut oils
These are likely to contain quite concentrated amounts of omega-6. It takes a great many nuts to produce a small amount of oil and the oil will not contain the whole package of nutrients that a complete nut possesses.

## Peanuts and peanut butter
Peanuts are not true nuts. They are legumes, are 53 per cent fat (mostly 'good' monounsaturated) and are extremely fattening. A cupful of peanuts contains more than 560 calories (a lot!). They also contain 5,000 times more omega-6 than omega-3. On the positive side peanuts contain fibre, protein, 'good' fat and many other nutrients, including antioxidants, which may protect against the inflammatory effect of omega-6.

Peanut butter, the organic brands with no added fat or sugar, is made of peanuts, sometimes roasted, that are ground together to form a paste. Unsurprisingly, peanut butter possesses the good and bad qualities of peanuts and therefore should be eaten in moderation. 'Reduced-fat' peanut butter may have something added to replace the fat – often high fructose corn syrup.

## Chestnuts
These are different to other nuts as they have a sweetish taste and no crunch. Chestnuts are low in fat. They contain starch and protein and are a source of beneficial minerals, vitamins and fibre. Their starch content gives them a moderate GI of 60.

## Coconuts
A discussion of coconuts needs a section to itself as there are highly divided opinions about the health benefits (or otherwise)

of eating coconut and coconut-based products. The disagreements all boil down to the dreaded 's' word: *saturated* fat.

Coconuts come from a type of palm and are quite different to tree nuts. The liquid inside a coconut is called water. Coconut cream is made from the meat, which is the thick white lining inside a coconut shell. Coconut milk is made from grated coconut meat and water (it can also be made at home from packs of creamed coconut). Coconut oil is a fat extracted from the meat. Coconut flour is dried coconut meat, in powdered form. These products all contain high levels of saturated fat.

Coconut adds flavour and nutrients to meals. It is rich in lauric acid – a substance that boosts the immune system. It is high in fibre, has a low GI (the GL of coconut meat is 5) and contains low levels of omega-6. Coconut oil is 87 per cent saturated fat and all coconut products are very high in calories. A cup of coconut milk contains 445 calories and 48g of saturated fat, although this can be reduced by using 'lite' coconut milk. Coconut flour contains high levels of protein and fibre and can reduce the glycaemic response to cakes and pastry. Dried coconut flakes often have added sugar.

| Product | Per cent fat |
|---|---|
| Coconut milk | 24 |
| Coconut milk, lite (reduced fat) | 10–14 according to variety |
| Coconut flour | 20 |

Whether high consumption of coconut-based products increases damaging blood cholesterol levels and therefore heart disease is still unresolved. Plant-based saturated fat has a different biochemical composition to the saturated fat found in food from animal sources. The countries that traditionally use coconut in their cooking usually combine it with a lot of vegetables and little or no meat – some researchers suggest that this is why the population in these countries remains healthy.

## Coconut oil

This is solid at room temperature and is sold in jars. It is 90 per cent saturated fat but half of this fat is lauric acid and there are known health benefits connected to this. The body uses lauric acid to fight viruses and bacteria. But the research that has established these benefits has all been short term. As yet there are no long-term studies into how coconut oil affects health.

## Coconut milk

Used to make delicious curries. Coconut milk has a low GI (41), the levels of omega-6 are low, the calorie count is high. Fat-reduced coconut milk contains significantly less fat and usually has much the same texture and taste, though brands vary.

## COOKING OILS

'Canola oil, sunflower oil, corn oil, olive oil, peanut oil – they are all sources of good heart healthy fat. Use them in place of butter.'

'Don't be fooled by the marketing. Don't buy these non-traditional non-healthy food-like substances.'

Google the question 'Which vegetable oil should I buy?' and you could come up with either of these answers. But how can there be such opposing opinions about vegetable oils? The answer is simple. It is a continuation of the ongoing fat controversy – which are the good fats? – with the same conflicting and sometimes extreme views.

Vegetable oil is the name given to any oil product derived from any plant. The oil may come from the fruit, seed, leaves or roots of the plant. A few oils can be cold-pressed – a method that involves minimal processing. But most oils are processed, as undesirable trace elements would otherwise make the oil bitter, over-pungent or too dark.

Different vegetable oils contain different ratios of saturated, monounsaturated and polyunsaturated fats and there seems to be agreement on both sides that oils high in monounsaturated fat are good for the heart. They help to lower 'bad' cholesterol and raise 'good' cholesterol levels in the blood. Oil marketed in the UK as a vegetable oil may be a blend of several oils or it may be rapeseed oil – the label will tell. Oils high in monounsaturated fat have a much longer shelf-life than other oils – this is because they are less prone to oxidisation than the polyunsaturated oils. All oils are high in calories.

So far, so good. Now for the disagreements. Vegetable oils with a high level of monounsaturated and polyunsaturated fat are the good oils. This is the traditional view. These oils help to improve blood cholesterol levels and so help to prevent heart disease. They are 'heart healthy'. But the writers who question this point out that a person is unlikely to eat a bowl of (as an example) sunflower seeds. Yet modern food technology has made it possible for them to consume the equivalent of a large amount of sunflower seeds by using sunflower oil. They are then eating the seeds in a far more concentrated form than nature intended.

These writers argue that the vegetable oils that are highly processed and contain a high level of polyunsaturated fat are very bad for you due to the chemical composition of polyunsaturated fats – substances that did not exist in our diet until the early 1900s, when new chemical processes made their manufacture possible. Two particular anxieties are:

1. That these oils are made largely from seeds – rapeseed, corn, sunflower etc. – and their oils cannot be extracted just by pressing. They have to undergo an intense and prolonged manufacturing process involving heat and treatment with chemical additives. At the end of this process some vegetable oils have to be deodorised to mask their highly unpleasant smell. Consequently, these vegetable oils are among the most chemically altered foods in our modern diet.

2. That vegetable oils, particularly those made from seeds and nuts, contain high levels of omega-6 fatty acids and low levels of omega-3. This causes an imbalance. Too much omega-6

can cause inflammation which, in turn, can cause a range of chronic ill-health and disease. It is estimated that a tablespoon of processed vegetable oil contains around 14g of omega-6. This is a lot – far more than the amount of omega-6 found in a quarter-cup of mixed nuts.

These issues may not have attracted much general attention but they are widely covered on the web, in food and health magazines, and in the BMJ where an American research team have recently published on the subject. In their conclusion they wrote: 'Advice to substitute polyunsaturated fats for saturated fats is a key component of worldwide dietary guidelines for coronary heart risk reduction. However, clinical benefits of the most abundant polyunsaturated fatty acid, omega-6 linoleic acid, have not been established.'[8] As yet, no definitive answers have been given, but this is an issue that is not going to go away.

## A look at three popular vegetable oils

*Canola oil*, a rapeseed oil, is marketed as being exceptionally healthy. Historically, rape oil was not made for human consumption as it contained a highly toxic acid but in the 1970s Canadian scientists developed a new variety of rapeseed by crossing it with a type of mustard plant. The oil obtained from this was called Canola (Canada Oil Low Acid). European rapeseed oil is now made from the same hybrid plant. Canola oil has very low saturated fat and very high monounsaturated fat levels and is the end product of a long complex chemical process during which the oil is exposed to high temperatures. Cold-pressed and/or organic rapeseed oil does not go through the same industrial process but, unfortunately, most rapeseed oils *are* made using the industrial processing method.

*Sunflower oil* is produced from sunflower seeds. It is light in taste and colour, has high vitamin E content and is a combination of

[8] 2013; 346:e8707 – Use of dietary linoleic acid for secondary prevention of coronary heart disease and death: evaluation of recovered data from the Sydney Diet Heart Study and updated meta-analysis. Lead researcher, C. E. Ramsden.

mono- and polyunsaturated fats with low saturated fat levels. The plant has been modified to produce different types of oil – high in oleic or linoleic acid. Sunflower oil is used extensively in the food and catering industry as it is tolerant of very high cooking and frying temperatures. It is mostly extracted through a chemical process. The high oleic variety contains very low levels of omega-6.

*Olive oil* is minimally processed. It has high levels of monounsaturated fat (mostly oleic acid) and antioxidants. Extra-virgin oil is the least processed. It is labelled as cold-pressed, which means that the oil is obtained by pressing and grinding the olives. Virgin comes from the second pressing. Pure olive oil has a degree of filtering and refining; extra light has undergone extensive processing (see Appendix 1 for more information about oil).

**Which is the right oil?**
All cooking oils are a mixture of saturated, monounsaturated and polyunsaturated fats. There is no definitive answer to the 'which one is best?' question but indications are that the oils high in heart-healthy monounsaturated fats are the better choice, although coconut oil may need to be treated as a special case – some writers commend it as the healthiest oil of all!

It is known that oils high in mono fats help to reduce cholesterol levels in the blood and lower the risk of heart disease and stroke. Most oils are highly processed and this may affect polyunsaturated fats in an unfavourable way. Only a few types – olive, peanut,

| Oil type | % omega-6 | % omega-3 | % monounsat. fat | % sat. fat |
|----------|-----------|-----------|------------------|------------|
| Coconut oil | 2 | 0 | 7 | 91 |
| Corn oil | 54 | 0 | 25 | 13 |
| Flaxseed oil | 18 | 57 | 16 | 9 |
| Olive oil | 8 | 1 | 77 | 14 |
| Peanut oil | 33 | 0 | 48 | 19 |
| Rapeseed oil | 20 | 9 | 62 | 6 |
| Sunflower oil* | 65 | 0 | 20 | 11 |
| *But high oleic sunflower oil contains only 4 per cent of omega-6. | | | | |

sunflower, coconut and rapeseed – can be cold-pressed and, because the yield on them is low, oils made this way are expensive.

As the previous chart shows, some vegetable oils contain very high amounts of omega-6. All oils are high in calories.

## ALCOHOL

The consensus of medical opinion regarding alcohol seems to contain good news for those who drink moderately. People with diabetes can continue to consume alcohol so long as the generally accepted guidelines are followed. Indeed, a review of the research surrounding diabetes and alcohol actually seems to suggest that moderate consumption of alcohol, particularly red wine, is good for you (although there are a few studies that query this finding). Most studies define moderate alcohol consumption as one to three units a day.

People may be surprised by this, believing that beer in particular contains a lot of sugar. However, many alcoholic drinks have virtually no carbohydrates in them. Beer is made with malted barley which, when brewed, turns into maltose. This is a sugar which is then converted into alcohol and the beer this produces contains little or no sugar. Beer is high in calories, not because of sugar but due to its alcohol. The same is true of dry wines, which contain virtually no sugar. Again, it is the alcohol that gives wine its calories. However, sweet and fortified wines do contain residual sugar. The GI of beer and wine cannot be measured as it would involve giving test subjects very large amounts of alcohol to drink over a very short time. What is known is that beer contains more residual carbohydrate than wine but, at around 12g per 350ml, this is still very low compared to other food items.

What beer and wine *are* high in are calories. Bitter, ale and stout contain 180–230 calories per pint. Bottled beers with 'light' in their name contain 90–100 calories. A medium glass of red wine contains 130 calories.

Alcohol often stimulates appetite. In other words, one or two beers can make some people long for a curry or a fry-up and researchers now believe they know why. Food after alcohol looks more appealing and this can interfere with appetite-control processes in the brain.

**Drinking alcohol is unsafe for people who have diabetic complications**, such as nerve damage or diabetic eye disease. For these people even moderate alcohol consumption may carry health risks as it can worsen these conditions. People who have diabetic complications or who are insulin users must always ask for professional guidance relating to their specific situation.

## CONCLUSION

Foods which 'might be okay' tend to include the contentious ones, their contentiousness usually referring back to the fat question. There is still scientific uncertainty about whether saturated fat and polyunsaturated fats are good or bad for you, but because some nuts and vegetable oils contain high levels of these fats then consumers really have to weigh up the evidence themselves. To be on the safe side they may decide to use less vegetable oil, to use different vegetable oils or to wait and see what the researchers tell us next. Alcohol is contentious for another reason. It is a two-faced substance: taken in moderation a tonic (perhaps), taken to excess, a poison.

---

**FOODS WHICH MIGHT BE OKAY: SUMMARY**

Nuts contain valuable nutrients but should be considered a treat. A diet with too many nuts can upset the balance between omega-3 and omega-6.

Coconuts contain high levels of saturated fat. There is disagreement as to whether this makes them a risk to heart health. All coconut products are high in calories.

Most cooking oils are highly processed. The oils high in monounsaturated oils may be the better choice. All oils are high in calories.

One tablespoon of processed vegetable oil contains a lot of omega-6. Use of processed vegetable oil is probably the main cause for the imbalance between omega-3 and omega-6 in our modern diet.

Moderate consumption of alcohol may be good for the heart. This does not apply to fortified or sweet dessert wines. All alcohol is high in calories.

---

# 2

## Eating Out

So, you've been looking forward to a meal out for ages. But where to go? First choice might be the local pub, and they may do a good steak there, but the chips or jacket potato that goes with it is not so good and the puddings are so tempting when everyone else is having one . . . Fast-food restaurants offer white-bun burger and chips and sugar-laden drinks; clearly not a good choice. Will Chinese be better? They certainly use a lot of vegetables but the white sticky rice, noodles and sauces that go with them may undo the good work that the vegetables are doing. Traditional fish and chips (fish well battered)? Oh dear, no. The Italian restaurant then: pasta has a medium GI, so will that be a better choice? Perhaps, but Italian restaurants may use fresh pasta (= rapid sugar spike), the amount of pasta in a portion is very large, and pizzas are notorious for what they do to your blood glucose level.

So what does that leave us? Clear soups, salads with lean meat or non-battered fish, grilled chicken, simple roasts with plenty of vegetables but only a small helping of potato – these might be on the menu of a good pub or restaurant. Indian, Turkish and Greek restaurants may offer more alternatives. Indian meals are often vegetarian and side-dishes of lentils and chick-peas can reduce the impact of high-GI food. Greek and Turkish restaurants offer mezes, stews and kebab-type dishes that are often low GI (but maybe not moussaka and definitely not baklava!). Spanish-style tapas restaurants are fun and offer small dishes, often vegetable-based and turned into something delicious. (But paellas and patatas bravas are best avoided.)

And, whichever the style of restaurant, keep portion sizes moderate.

# 10

## Is This the Perfect Meal?

Scientists from an independent UK food research agency drew up the 'Perfect Meal' shortlist. The researchers examined the health claims of over 4,000 food products and reduced them to 222 judged to have real merit. From these, the scientists produced their perfect menu.

*Starter*: fresh and smoked salmon terrine with a mixed leaf salad with extra-virgin olive oil dressing and a high-fibre multigrain bread roll.

*Main course*: chicken casserole with lentils and mixed vegetables.

*Pudding*: yoghurt-based blancmange with walnuts and sugar-free caramel-flavoured sauce.

# 11

## Afterword From a Diabetes Survivor

It was lucky for me when my wife determined to cut through the myths and contradictions surrounding diabetes and find out what she could safely feed me. And, you know, it's not all dull and boring stuff. Although some meals have been quietly fed to the dog I have discovered new foods and flavours. And it's reassuring to know that what you're eating is good for you as well as satisfying to your appetite. So, a few years after diagnosis, I'm still here and life is good.

In fact, I've never felt so well since they told me I was ill!

Peter

# APPENDIX 1

## Key Nutritional Terms

### WHAT IS INSULIN RESISTANCE?

Insulin is a powerful hormone. It does many jobs in the body, one being to make the body's cells take up glucose and use what is needed as energy. Any surplus is stored. In modern society nearly everybody produces a surplus. In other words they eat too much. People who lead an incredibly active life may turn all the food they eat into energy but most people do not burn it all off and the body has to store it somewhere.

After being eaten, carbohydrates turn into glucose. Although glucose provides the energy for muscles to work, it has to be converted into energy before it can do this. The pancreas, aware somehow that there is lots of glucose in the blood, secretes insulin. This allows the glucose to enter the cells and muscles of the body, where it is either used for immediate energy needs or stored in the form of glycogen. But in some people the cells become resistant to insulin and the glucose is unable to enter the cells. However, the pancreas still 'knows' that there is too much glucose in these people's blood so it produces even more insulin. There may now be an excess of insulin as well as glucose in the bloodstream. Things have got badly out of balance.

Without medical intervention blood glucose levels remain high because the body cells can no longer receive it. This thickens the blood. It clogs arteries and binds with other compounds to form harmful end products. This increases the risk of heart disease and other complications. Insulin levels in the blood may also remain high and this also is dangerous. High levels of insulin also contribute to heart disease and other diseases. Eventually the pancreas exhausts itself and becomes unable to produce any more insulin.

What is the cause of this? Insulin resistance seems to be partly genetic but body weight is a major factor, and reducing weight, even by just 10 per cent, and aiming for a normal body mass index (20–25) will reduce insulin resistance and improve blood glucose levels.

## WHAT IS PROTEIN?

Proteins are large molecules made from smaller units called amino acids. They are part of every cell, tissue and organ in the human body. These body proteins are constantly being broken down and need to be replaced. The protein that we eat is turned into amino acids and this is used to replace these lost body proteins. There are twenty-two types of amino acid. The human body needs all of them and is able to produce most of them by itself. However, there are eight amino acids that the human body cannot produce. Foods that contains all eight of these are called 'complete proteins' and come from animal products like meat, cheese, eggs and fish. Proteins that do not include all eight of these essential amino acids are called 'incomplete proteins' and come from plant products like fruit, vegetables, grain and nuts. Vegetarians have to combine 'incomplete proteins' in order to get a complete range of amino acids. This is why they are advised to eat beans and bread together, or lentils and rice. Meat- and dairy-eaters get a complete range of amino acids.

The recommended daily protein requirement for an adult is approximately 0.8g of protein per kilogram of body weight for an average person. People involved in heavy work or sport may need slightly more.

Cooked red meat is 27–35 per cent protein; beans, nuts and lentils are around 25 per cent; grains are 10 per cent.

### Some examples of amounts of protein in food

> 3oz/75g of meat contains 21g of protein
> 1 cup of dry beans contains 16g of protein

8oz/200ml yoghurt contains 11g of protein
1 cup of milk contains 8g of protein

These examples show that people on a normal balanced diet are unlikely to be at risk of not eating enough protein. In fact, most people eat much more.

## WHAT IS INFLAMMATION?

Inflammation, the body's response to injury or illness, is part of the body's immune response system. It is the body's attempt to rid itself of harmful stimuli so that the healing process can begin. The symptoms of inflammation that go with an external injury such as an ingrowing toenail are heat, redness and swelling, and these feelings, uncomfortable as they are, have a purpose. Heat (increased blood flow) brings healing agents (eicosanoids) to the site of the injury and the swelling indicates that these agents are doing their work of breaking down the damaged tissue and starting to rebuild with healthy tissue.

The problems begin when inflammation becomes chronic. It causes further inflammation and becomes self-perpetuating as more inflammation is created in response to the existing inflammation. Infections, wounds etc. cannot heal without inflammation. However, chronic inflammation can eventually lead to many diseases and conditions.

The healing hormones produced by the body regulate the immune system. There are two types – pro- and anti-inflammatory and both are needed, in proper balance. Pro-inflammatory hormones come from eating food rich in omega-6; the anti- ones come from food rich in omega-3.

### Diabetes and inflammation

It is known that there is a link between obesity and diabetes, but how does it work? Researchers have discovered that white blood cells combine with fat cells and release inflammatory chemicals called cytokines which interfere with the ability of body cells to take up insulin. This explains why patients who have gastric band surgery may see their Type 2 symptoms disappear. The fat producing the inflammatory chemicals is lost and this reverses their insulin resistance.

## WHAT IS A CALORIE?

A calorie is a unit of energy. By definition one calorie is the energy it takes to raise the temperature of 1g of water by 1 degree Celsius. When talked about in relation to food the term kilocalories is used. Calories equal energy, and an average human body needs at least 1,000 calories to have sufficient fuel just to keep the key essential organs working. Extra energy is required to actually do anything (for example, move around). If a person consumes more calories than he or she requires they will eventually gain weight. General guidelines are that men need 2,500 and women need 2,000 calories per day. Of these calories, 30 per cent should come from fat (at least two-thirds of which should be unsaturated).

## WHAT IS GOOD CHOLESTEROL?
## WHAT IS BAD CHOLESTEROL?

Cholesterol is a waxy substance produced by the liver and found in certain food derived from animals. Among other things it is needed to make vitamin D, to maintain body cells and to create bile (needed to digest fat). However, a human liver produces about 1,000mg of cholesterol a day and the cholesterol provided by burgers and bacon is an addition to this. About 85 per cent of blood cholesterol is produced by the body. The other 15 per cent comes from diet.

Some people have higher than normal cholesterol levels and the prime cause of this is thought to be genetic. Other causes are high blood pressure, a fatty diet, stress and obesity. Dietary cholesterol is not a factor but a diet high in saturated fat is because the liver has to produce more cholesterol in order to digest the fat. The more saturated fat we eat the more cholesterol we make.

Cholesterol and other fats cannot dissolve in water. This means that they cannot dissolve in blood. To move through the bloodstream they have to attach themselves to body proteins and these form lipoproteins. High-density lipoproteins (HDLs) are sometimes called 'good cholesterol' because they actually remove cholesterol from the blood vessels and take it back to the liver, from where it is eventually eliminated. Unfortunately, most cholesterol forms low-density lipoproteins (LDLs). These are called 'bad cholesterol' because they clog up the blood vessels and restrict the flow of blood.

Foods containing soluble fibre (fruit, vegetables, oats and legumes) reduce levels of LDLs. They do this by reducing the absorption of cholesterol into the bloodstream. Other foods that reduce 'bad' cholesterol include foods high in monounsaturated fat (olives, olive oil, oily fish, avocado). But, unlike vegetables, most of these foods are also high in calories. The most efficient way to naturally reduce blood cholesterol is to eat a vegetable-rich diet.

## WHAT IS BODY MASS INDEX?

This formula became popular in 1972 when a researcher found that the BMI was a method of showing the ratio between body weight and height. This was of interest because obesity was beginning to emerge as a problem in Western society. The BMI gives a simple figure to a person's fatness or thinness. One of the reasons for its use is that doctors can talk about overweight (or underweight) objectively. Uncomfortable words like 'fat' do not have to be used.

| BMI | Classification |
|---|---|
| Under 20 | Underweight |
| 20–25 | Normal |
| 25–29.9 | Overweight |
| 30+ | Obese |

BMI is calculated by dividing your weight in kilograms by the square of your height in centimetres. Or by dividing your weight in pounds by the square of your height in inches, then multiplying by 703. For example, a 5ft 4in (64 inches) woman weighing 126 pounds would have a BMI of 21.6 (i.e. $126 / 64^2 \times 703$).

BMI values can be calculated quickly and cheaply. However, they do not take into account things like muscularity, bone density or frame-size. Thus, athletes may be considered 'obese' because of increased muscle-weight, while elderly people may be considered 'underweight' because of reduced bone density.

## WHAT ARE ANTIOXIDANTS?
These are nutrients or enzymes that counteract the damaging effects of oxidation in animal tissue. Oxidation is caused by free radicals. These are the molecules responsible for ageing and tissue damage. Oxidation is a factor in many diseases, including cancer; antioxidants can help to prevent this. The antioxidants found in vegetables are called flavonoids.

## WHAT ARE FLAVONOIDS?
Flavonoids, or bioflavonoids, are antioxidants that are found in many fruit and vegetables and give them their bright colours. Aside from their antioxidant effect, eating foods containing flavonoids is beneficial because it triggers the production of natural enzymes in the body that fight disease. Fruit and vegetables that contain high amounts of flavonoids are those with deep or bright colours. These include all red, black and blue berries, citrus fruit, broccoli, tomatoes, red beans, soy, red wine and tea. Only a small amount of flavonoids need be consumed for their health benefits to start working. Flavanols are antioxidants that are particularly concentrated in cocoa beans and give similar health benefits.

Flavonoids are sometimes referred to as vitamin P.

## MORE ABOUT OIL
UK supermarkets now give a huge amount of shelf space to olive oil and upmarket brands are very expensive. But what is a 'good'

olive oil and how is a good one distinguished from a bad one? Traditionally, the best extra-virgin oils come from Italy and are not refined or blended. The initials DOP on the label (translated as Protected Designation of Origin) gives a guarantee of quality and origin. Olive oil experts say that a 'good' oil should have layers of complex flavours. It should taste slightly bitter and may make your throat burn. Oils that are bland or slightly sweet are considered inferior. Expensive extra-virgin oils will have the date of harvest on the label and possibly the farm of origin or maker.

The cheaper bottles of olive oil are blends. They can be a mix of olive varieties, harvested and stored in different places at different times. Some food experts claim that a lot of so-called extra-virgin oil is refined and therefore fraudulent. A journalist investigating this believes that olive oil fraud is lucrative, widespread and difficult to prove.

Traditionally, olive oil has come from the Mediterranean countries but Australia, South Africa, Chile and America are all now developing their own olive oil industries.

All types of olive oil have the health benefits associated with monounsaturated fat. Extra-virgin is made from the best-quality olives and is the least processed so may contain more health-giving nutrients than others.

Cold-pressed oil is any oil that is produced by pressing the seed, grain or nut that produces it, at low heat. Introducing heat to the process reduces the colour and nutrient value of the oil. It also greatly increases the yield and this is the reason why cold-pressed oils are so expensive. The product is ground to produce a paste; the paste is then slowly stirred and this causes the oil to separate. More oil can be extracted by heating the paste.

Cold-pressed rapeseed oil, now being produced by UK farmers, is sometimes referred to as the English olive oil. It contains half the saturated fat of olive oil.

# APPENDIX 2

## Recipes

**RECIPE NOTES**

**Cardamom:** this gives a lovely flavour to both savoury and sweet dishes. It is easy to find cardamom pods but extracting and then crushing the seeds is tedious. Ground cardamom can be bought online.

**Cheese sauce:** this is usually based on a cooked white sauce. Here are two alternatives:
1. Mix a carton of ricotta cheese with a carton of single cream and some grated low-fat Cheddar. 2. Less rich. Mix a carton of crème fraîche with a splash of milk, some grain mustard and grated low-fat Cheddar.

**Coconut milk:** to make 400ml, dissolve 135g of coconut cream in 400ml of boiling water. To make 150ml, dissolve 50g coconut cream in 150ml boiling water.

**De-skinning:** cut *peppers* into quarters and de-seed. Grill until the skin is black and blistering. Wrap in foil, leave to cool in their own steam then de-skin when cool. Cover *tomatoes* with boiling water. Leave to cool then stab with a knife and de-skin.

**Dried beans:** these must be soaked overnight or for 6–8 hours. They must then be brought to the boil in a pan of fresh water and simmered for 2–3 hours, until soft. Allow 50g of beans per person. **Dried chick-peas** also need overnight soaking but do not take so long to cook.

**Lentils:** different-coloured lentils taste similar but cook up differently. Red lentils cook quickly but do not hold their shape.

Brown and green lentils contain more fibre, hold their shape and give more texture. French or Puy lentils have a slight peppery taste and are the connoisseur's choice of lentils.

**Olives** are used in some of the recipes. 'Pitted Dry Black Olives with Herbs' from Crespo are plump, juicy and moist. Too salty to eat on their own, they are good for use in recipes and can be purchased in multiple packs online.

**Parmesan** is the name of an extra-hard cheese that originated in Italy. Best, and most expensive, is Parmigiano-Reggiano – produced only in specific cities in northern Italy. Other countries also produce hard cheeses – for example, Reggianito comes from Argentina. Parmesan cheese always contains calf rennet (a stomach enzyme) so is not okay for vegetarians. Vegetarian pasta cheese is made with cow's milk and vegetarian rennet.

**Ras el hanout:** a spice blend of cardamom, clove, cinnamon, chilli, coriander, cumin, nutmeg and turmeric.

**Spinach:** 450g of fresh spinach is the equivalent of 170g frozen. Heat frozen spinach in a heavy saucepan with a knob of butter and a little milk or cream. Use lumps of frozen spinach to thicken stews and casseroles.

**Sweating:** the gentle frying of chopped vegetables in a little oil or butter preliminary to further cooking.

**Tinned tomatoes:** additives in the canning process can make tomatoes salty or acidic. The San Marzano brand are naturally sweeter and are harvested when ripe. Two other well-thought-of brands are Red Gold and Pomi.

**Yoghurt sauce:** mix 200g thick yoghurt with 2 tbsp olive oil and 2 tbsp chopped mint.

# BREAKFAST

## PORRIDGE

*Instant porridge is usually made in the microwave. It has added sugar, has had most of its nutrients stripped away and has a very high GI. Real porridge, made with jumbo or rolled oats, is far more nutritious. Brands seem to cook up with differing degrees of stickiness; Irish, or steel-cut oats, are said to produce a breakfast that is least sticky. Cook porridge in a non-stick saucepan to avoid difficult washing-up.*

**Flavourings for porridge:** try vanilla extract; cinnamon and/or nutmeg; ground cardamom mixed with a crushed clove; dried fruit; fresh berries. A pear or apple grated into the oats during cooking will sweeten and reduce the need for sugar. The amount of liquid used to cook the oats will vary according to whether people like their porridge thick or runny.

# MUESLI
## (10 SERVINGS)

*The amounts can be varied and other things added – flaked bran, flaked almonds, barley or rye flakes etc. Experiment and find the recipe that best suits you but go easy on the dried fruit and do not use dried dates as their GI value is very high.*

750g oat flakes
240g mixed nuts (not salted)
120g pumpkin seeds
120g sunflower seeds
120g raisins
120g chopped apricots

Mix everything together and store in an airtight container.

# PORRIDGE ON THE HOB
## (2 SERVINGS)

60g oats
2–3 cups milk
1 apple, grated
a few sultanas
1 tsp cinnamon (optional)
1 banana, sliced/berries
1–2 tsp brown sugar
single cream (optional)

Put the oats, milk, grated apple and sultanas into a saucepan and bring to the boil. Simmer, add the cinnamon and stir until porridge thickens. Stir in the banana or berries, add sugar and serve with a swirl of single cream.

# OATY PANCAKES
### (ABOUT 10 SMALL PANCAKES)

*Whizz up oat flakes in a food processor to make oatmeal.*

30g oatmeal
10g wholemeal flour
1 egg
1 tsp baking powder
1 tsp vanilla extract
$\frac{1}{2}$ tsp cinnamon
50–60 ml milk
oil for frying

Mix everything together – it does not need to be too liquid. Heat some oil to a high temperature in a frying pan or griddle. Pour in 1 tablespoon of mixture at a time. Confine or flatten into pancake shapes. Cook one side then turn and cook the other. Serve warm with honey, maple syrup, jam etc. or with a teaspoon of crème fraîche and fresh berries. (If pancakes are too irregular in shape and need to look neater, cut into a round shape with a scone cutter.)

# SOUPS

*A healthy alternative to a sandwich-based lunch. A big saucepanful, made with lentils or split peas, can provide lunch for several days.*

## MULLIGATAWNY SOUP
### (4 SERVINGS)

*Mulligatawny, from the Tamil* milagu tanni, *means 'pepper water'.*

200g red lentils
1–2 small potatoes, diced
1 litre chicken or vegetable stock
200g uncooked chicken pieces
1 small piece fresh ginger, peeled
oil, for frying
4 cloves garlic, chopped finely
1 onion, chopped
1/2 tsp each of cumin, turmeric, cayenne pepper and ground coriander
2 tbsp lemon juice
Marmite or Oxo cube (optional)
fresh coriander or parsley for garnish
1 tsp garam masala

Bring the lentils and potatoes to a boil in the stock and then simmer for 30 minutes. Mash into a purée with a potato masher. De-skin the chicken and cut into bite-sized pieces. Grate the ginger. Fry the chicken for 2 minutes in a little oil, then add the ginger, garlic and onion and sweat gently. Add all the spices to the meat and cook gently for 5 minutes. Season well and add the lemon juice. Add some Marmite or Oxo if the soup needs extra flavour. Stir in the lentil/potato purée and warm thoroughly. Garnish with chopped coriander.

# SWEET POTATO AND COCONUT SOUP

(4 SERVINGS)

1 large sweet potato, peeled
1 green chilli, de-seeded
1 onion, chopped
oil, for frying
2–3 small tomatoes, de-skinned and chopped
some fresh coriander
400ml tin low-fat coconut milk
400ml stock
salt and cayenne pepper

Cut the sweet potato into small chunks, then boil until soft. Drain. Cut the chilli into very fine pieces and sweat with the onion in a little oil for a few minutes. Add the tomatoes and cook for another minute. Whizz the vegetables up in a blender with the coriander (add a little liquid if necessary). Put back in the saucepan and add the coconut milk and stock. Simmer, do not allow to boil. Add salt and a pinch of cayenne pepper to taste.

# CREAM OF MUSHROOM SOUP
(6–8 SERVINGS)

*Optional – use some white wine to make up the stock.*

2 onions, chopped
1 clove garlic, chopped
85g butter
500g mushrooms, chopped
parsley, chopped
plain flour to thicken
1 litre stock
small carton of single cream

Gently cook the onions and garlic in melted butter, then add the mushrooms and parsley and cook until soft. Stir the flour into the mixture, cook for a minute or two, then add the stock. Stir and bring to the boil, then season well and simmer for 10 minutes. Whizz the soup in a blender, return to the pan and stir in the cream. Heat through and serve.

# SPLIT GREEN PEA SOUP WITH BACON

## (4 SERVINGS)

*A thick hearty soup.*

4 bacon rashers, cut into small pieces
1 large onion, chopped
2 cloves garlic, chopped
180g green split peas
1 litre chicken or vegetable stock
2 cups cold water
2 tbsp lemon juice
sweet paprika

Fry the bacon pieces then set aside. Gently fry the onion and garlic in bacon juice until transparent. Add the split peas and stir. Add the stock and water. Bring to the boil, then simmer for 30–40 minutes, until the liquid has been absorbed and the split peas are soft. Stir in the lemon juice. Whizz up in a blender. Add more water or stock to get to the desired consistency. Cut the bacon into shreds and stir into the soup. Sprinkle with paprika before serving.

# CURRIED SALMON CHOWDER

## (4 SERVINGS)

1 onion
2 tsp green Thai curry paste
500ml vegetable stock
55g creamed coconut, cut into small pieces
2–3 small potatoes
2 salmon fillets
220ml single cream
50ml white wine
chopped parsley

Sweat the onion until it is transparent, then stir in the curry paste. Add the stock and creamed coconut. Simmer and stir until the coconut is dissolved. Dice the potatoes into bite-sized pieces, add to the soup and simmer until cooked, 8–10 minutes. Gently coax and pull the skin off the salmon and then cut the fish into bite-sized pieces. Add the cream and a generous splash of wine to the soup, then add the salmon and simmer gently for 2–3 minutes only. Serve garnished with parsley.

# CURRIED CREAM OF CAULIFLOWER SOUP
## (4 SERVINGS)

*Use green Thai curry paste to retain the pale colour of the cauliflower.*

1 onion
1 tbsp olive oil
3 tsp medium curry paste
1 small cauliflower, separated into florets
a little plain flour
500ml stock
400ml tin low-fat coconut milk

Chop the onion finely, then sweat in the oil. Stir in the curry paste and cauliflower. When the florets are well coated, sprinkle with flour and stir until the flour is cooked. Add sufficient stock to cover the cauliflower, bring to the boil and simmer until florets are soft. Whizz in a blender, then return to the saucepan and add the coconut milk. Season to taste. Simmer to bring back to the required temperature.

# PÂTÉS AND DIPS

*Serve with vegetable crudités, radishes and black olives, sourdough toast, wholemeal pitta bread cut into fingers etc.*

## SMOKED MACKEREL PÂTÉ

### (4–6 SERVINGS)

2 smoked mackerel
140g ricotta or low-fat cream cheese
140g Greek yoghurt
juice of 1 lemon

Whizz everything together in a blender and season to taste.

## SMOKED SALMON PÂTÉ

### (4–6 SERVINGS)

*A rich pâté – a good starter with squares of toasted sourdough and a salad garnish.*

100g smoked salmon
80g softened butter
2 tbsp Greek yoghurt
chopped chives or spring onion tops

Whizz everything together in a blender and season to taste.

# TUNA PÂTÉ

(4–6 SERVINGS)

1 small tin tuna (in oil), drained
50g soft butter
juice and zest of half a lemon
1 tbsp olive oil
1 tbsp brandy
freshly ground black pepper

Whizz everything together in a blender. Add more oil if the mixture is too thick.

# MUSHROOM PÂTÉ

(4–6 SERVINGS)

1 small onion, chopped
1 clove garlic, chopped
2 tbsp olive oil
160g button mushrooms, sliced
salt and freshly ground black pepper
50g low-fat cream cheese
chopped parsley

Sweat the onion and garlic in the olive oil for a few minutes, then add the mushrooms with another drizzle of oil. Stir and gently cook for 8–10 minutes (this cooks the moisture out of the mushrooms without burning them). Season well, then tip into a blender with the cheese and parsley. Whizz until smooth. Season to taste.

# HUMMUS
(4–6 SERVINGS)

tin chick-peas or butter beans
2 tbsp low-fat Greek yoghurt
2 tbsp lemon juice
olive oil
1 level tbsp tahini paste (optional)
handful of chopped parsley

Drain and rinse the chick-peas. Season well and whizz in a food processor with the yoghurt and lemon juice. Add oil to the desired consistency. (Optional – add 1 level tbsp of tahini.) Sprinkle with chopped parsley before serving.

# FLAVOURED HUMMUS

*Lime and mint or thyme:* add juice and zest of one lime with chopped fresh mint or fresh thyme.

*Roasted red pepper:* grill and de-skin a red pepper, and whizz up with the mixture.

# CREAMY TUNA DIP

### (4–6 SERVINGS)

400g tin of tuna (in oil)
1 tin cannellini beans
1 carton low-fat cream cheese
handful of watercress, chopped
2 tbsp reduced-fat mayonnaise
2 tbsp reduced-fat Greek yoghurt
zest and juice of 1 lemon or lime
handful of chopped herbs (optional)

Whizz everything together in a blender.


# CREAMY PESTO DIP

### (4–6 SERVINGS)

*The amount of pesto to use depends on personal preference.*

1 carton low-fat cream cheese
1 tbsp low-fat Greek yoghurt
fresh pesto (see pesto recipe, page 122)
1 clove garlic, chopped

Whizz everything together in a blender.

# PEPPER AND WHITE BEAN DIP

(4–6 SERVINGS)

1 red pepper, de-skinned
1 tin cannellini beans, drained
1 tbsp olive oil
6 pitted black olives
2 tsp balsamic vinegar

Whizz everything together in a blender.


# TAPENADE

(4–6 SERVINGS)

200g black herby olives, de-stoned
1 clove garlic, chopped
1 tbsp capers, drained
4 anchovy fillets, drained
3–4 tbsp olive oil
juice of 1 lemon

Whizz everything together in a blender.

# STARTERS

## TAPENADE TOASTS WITH EGG AND GHERKIN
### (6–8 SERVINGS)

1 sourdough loaf cut into rounds and toasted
100g of tapenade
1 hard-boiled egg, thinly sliced
gherkins, sliced

Spread the toast with tapenade. Top some with a slice of hard-boiled egg, others with sliced gherkin.


## MUSHROOMS ON SOURDOUGH
### (6–8 SERVINGS)

*A tapas recipe from Spain.*
*This recipe does not work with big mushrooms.*

170g button mushrooms
1 tbsp olive oil
1 tsp dry sherry
a pinch of salt and black pepper
slices of sourdough bread
low-fat mayonnaise

Slice the mushrooms thinly. Heat the oil with the sherry, salt and pepper in a saucepan. Add the mushrooms, cover and cook on a very low heat until the mushrooms release their liquid. Spread the sourdough with mayonnaise. Top with the drained mushroom slices, then put under a preheated grill until the mayonnaise is bubbling. Serve immediately.

# RED PEPPER ROLLS WITH FETA

## (4 SERVINGS)

*These rolls can also be made with strips of aubergine that have been lightly sprayed with olive oil then grilled or roasted in the oven.*

2 red peppers, quartered lengthways
100g feta cheese
16 black herby olives, de-stoned
16 basil leaves, torn
1 tbsp pesto sauce
1 tbsp salad dressing

Grill and de-skin the peppers. Chop the feta and olives and mix together with the basil leaves. Pile some mixture on each pepper quarter, then roll up and secure with a cocktail stick. Whisk the pesto and salad dressing together and drizzle over the pepper rolls.

# PIEDMONTESE PEPPERS

(4 SERVINGS)

4 red peppers, halved lengthways
4 large tomatoes, de-skinned and halved
basil leaves, torn
4 cloves garlic, sliced
4 anchovies, chopped
olive oil

When halving the peppers cut through the stalk vertically in half so that each pepper has a piece of stalk attached. De-seed the peppers and place them in an oven-proof dish in a single layer. Scoop out the watery flesh from the centre of the tomatoes and put one tomato in each pepper half. Mix the basil leaves, garlic and anchovies with a little oil and fill each tomato with the anchovy mixture. Season with black pepper, then drizzle oil over each pepper and roast in a preheated oven at 180°C (gas mark 4) for 35 minutes. Serve warm with bread to mop up the juices.

# AVOCADO AND BACON IN A HOT DRESSING

(4 SERVINGS)

2 rashers of bacon
4 tbsp olive oil
2 tomatoes, de-skinned
3 tbsp red wine vinegar
4 tsp Dijon mustard
2 ripe avocados, peeled

Chop the bacon and fry in a little of the oil until slightly crisp. Chop the tomatoes, then add to the bacon with the vinegar, oil and mustard. Leave to bubble for a few minutes. Dice the avocados. Mix everything gently together and serve warm with bread to mop up the juice.

# PASTA SAUCES AND PASTA DISHES

*Serve with cooked pasta but remember that a healthy serving of pasta is no more than 40g uncooked. The GI of pasta is reduced if the pasta is allowed to cool and then reheated. An alternative to wheat-based spaghetti is vegetable spaghetti. A simple kitchen tool can be obtained that turns courgettes or carrots into spaghetti-like strands.*

## QUICK TOMATO SAUCE WITH BASIL
### (4 SERVINGS)

*A sauce that can be used with pasta dishes, stirred into a tin of beans or used as a sauce for meatballs. Make with fresh or tinned tomatoes.*

4–5 large tomatoes, de-skinned, or 1 tin tomatoes.
2 cloves garlic, crushed and chopped
1 onion, chopped
50g chopped basil
1 tsp oregano
1 tbsp olive oil
tomato paste (optional)

Chop the tomatoes. Sweat the garlic, onion and herbs in the oil. Add the tomatoes. Bring to the boil then simmer until the tomatoes are reduced and the sauce is thick – this will take about 20 minutes. Season and add more olive oil and/or a dollop of tomato paste, to taste. Whizz in a blender and add a little extra oil for a smooth sauce.

# LENTIL BOLOGNESE SAUCE

(4–6 SERVINGS)

1 onion, chopped
2 cloves garlic, crushed
2 carrots, grated
2 celery stalks, chopped
3 tbsp olive oil
150g red lentils
400g tin chopped tomatoes
3 tbsp tomato paste
800ml stock
fresh marjoram/thyme/oregano

Gently fry the onion, garlic, carrots and celery in the oil until soft. Add the lentils, tomatoes, tomato paste, stock and herbs. Season, then bring to the boil. Partially cover and simmer for 20 minutes until the sauce is thick and soft. Serve with spaghetti.

# MARINARA SAUCE

## (MAKES THE EQUIVALENT OF 3 TINS OF SAUCE)

*Invented by Neapolitan sailors after the introduction of the tomato to
Europe. Serve with pasta, beans, or use as a base for other dishes.
Best made with Chantenay carrots as they give the sauce
a pleasant sweetness.*

1 onion, finely chopped
2 cloves garlic, finely chopped
2 carrots, peeled and finely chopped
olive oil
several sprigs of fresh oregano
2 bay leaves
1/2 tsp salt
1/2 tsp crushed black peppercorns
450g fresh tomatoes, de-skinned and chopped, or 2 tins chopped
tomatoes

Sweat the onion, garlic and carrots in a little oil with the herbs,
salt and crushed peppercorns for 10 minutes. Add the tomatoes.
Bring to the boil, then simmer on a very low heat for 30 minutes.
Remove the bay leaves and stir in extra olive oil until the sauce
is thick and rich.

# PESTO SAUCE

*Traditionally made with pine nuts, this pesto recipe is more economical. The ratio of basil, cheese and oil is variable, according to taste. Quantities given here are for a mini electric food processor – they should be doubled for a standard-size processor. Pesto keeps well in the fridge or can be frozen – cubes of pesto can be frozen in an ice-tray for use later.*

50g raw (unsalted) cashew nuts or walnuts
½ clove garlic, chopped
100g basil
20–35g Parmesan, grated
100ml olive oil
freshly ground black pepper

Whizz up the nuts and garlic in a blender, then add everything else. Go lightly on the cheese as it can overpower.

# MAIN MEALS WITH PASTA

## MUSHROOM RAGU

### (4 SERVINGS)

*A ragu is a meat-based Italian sauce, served with pasta.
This recipe uses mushrooms and anchovies in place of meat,
and star anise gives it a distinctive flavour.*

4 anchovies, drained
1 onion, 1 carrot and 1 celery stick
2 tbsp olive oil
700g plain tomato sauce
50ml white wine
1 star anise
220g button mushrooms
50g butter
120g pasta, cooked
parsley, chopped
Parmesan, grated

Chop the anchovies. Chop the onion, carrot and celery and gently cook them with the anchovies in a little oil for 10 minutes. Add the tomato sauce, wine and star anise and simmer for 20 minutes – until reduced. Season. Slice the mushrooms and fry in a little butter or oil. Add the mushrooms to the sauce and gently heat though. Remove the star anise, serve with pasta and sprinkle with parsley and Parmesan.

# AUBERGINE RIGATONI

(4 SERVINGS)

450g small tomatoes, halved
1 aubergine, sliced
olive oil
2 cloves garlic, crushed in olive oil
120g penne or rigatoni, cooked
fresh basil, chopped
50g herby black olives, de-stoned and chopped
300g mozzarella, sliced thinly
Parmesan, grated

Drizzle the tomatoes with oil, brush the aubergine slices with oil, and bake the tomatoes and aubergine slices in a preheated oven at 180°C (gas mark 4) for 40 minutes. Mix the garlicy oil with the pasta and turn half the mixture into a baking dish. Scatter half the tomatoes over this, sprinkle the basil over the top, then add the olives and some slices of mozzarella. Season well. Lay the aubergine slices over the mixture, add the rest of the pasta and the remaining tomatoes and mozzarella. Top with Parmesan and bake in a preheated oven at 180°C (gas mark 4) for 20 minutes.

# MULTI-FLAVOURED LASAGNE

## (4–6 SERVINGS)

*A dish of lasagne can be a simple meal for two or it can be turned into
a multi-layered, multi-flavoured dish for a larger gathering.
This recipe uses a generous quantity of marinara or tomato sauce.
It needs to be cooked in a very deep baking dish to accommodate
its five different-flavoured layers.*

1 tub ricotta cheese
40ml single cream
100g Cheddar cheese, grated
450g small mushrooms, sliced
2 cloves garlic, peeled and crushed
plain flour to thicken
200ml milk
fresh or frozen spinach
100g mixed olives, de-stoned and chopped
200ml marinara (see page 121) or tomato sauce
sheets of wholemeal lasagne pasta

Mix the ricotta, cream and grated Cheddar together and put to
one side. Cook the mushrooms in a little olive oil with the garlic.
Season, then sprinkle the mushrooms with flour and stir to make
a paste. Cook for a minute then add milk or cream and bring to
the boil while still stirring to make a thinnish sauce. Put to one
side. Cook or defrost the spinach and squeeze out all the moisture.
Put to one side. Chop a generous amount of olives and put to one
side. With the marinara sauce these will be the five contrasting
layers that make up the lasagne.

Spread the marinara sauce over the bottom of the baking dish and
cover with a layer of pasta. Add the spinach and cover this layer with
more pasta. Then layer the mushroom mixture, cover with pasta,
then the olives, another layer of pasta and finish with the ricotta
mixture spread over the top. Bake in a preheated oven at 180°C (gas
mark 4) for 30–40 minutes.

# MAIN MEALS

## MAIN MEALS WITHOUT MEAT

### BAKED CAULIFLOWER CHEESE

(4–6 SERVINGS)

*This turns cauliflower cheese into a complete meal.*

1 cauliflower
4–6 small potatoes, sliced
50g wholemeal breadcrumbs
1 clove garlic, finely sliced
8 crushed black peppercorns
Parmesan, grated
2 tbsp melted butter or olive oil
500ml cheese sauce
500ml marinara sauce (see page 121)
¼ tsp chilli powder

Divide the cauliflower into smallish sections. Boil the potatoes and steam the cauliflower at the same time – do not overcook. Mix the breadcrumbs, garlic, crushed peppercorns and Parmesan with the butter or oil. Put the cauliflower into an oven-proof dish and place the potato slices among it. Pour the cheese sauce over and top with the breadcrumb mixture. Bake in a preheated oven at 170°C (between gas mark 3 and 4) for 30 minutes, until browned and bubbling. Warm the marinara sauce, add the chilli powder and stir well. When ready to serve, spoon the sauce onto the middle of each plate, spread it into a circle and place a serving of baked cauliflower in the middle.

# BEAN CASSEROLE

### (3–4 SERVINGS)

1 onion, chopped
2 cloves garlic, chopped
2 tbsp olive oil
1 tin kidney beans in chilli sauce
4 small potatoes, diced
a few small carrots, cut into chunks
1 green pepper, de-seeded and chopped
1 bean tin of white wine or stock
black pepper, to taste

Gently cook the onion and garlic in a little oil until soft. Mix everything together and cook as a casserole in a preheated oven at 150°C (gas mark 2) for 90 minutes (give it an occasional stir) or cook in a slow cooker on low for 4–5 hours.

# MUSHROOM STROGANOFF

## (4 SERVINGS)

*Choose big meaty mushrooms and slice them,
or use button mushrooms and halve them.*

1 large onion, sliced
4 celery sticks, chopped
2 cloves garlic, crushed and chopped
2 tbsp olive oil
2 tbsp butter
200g mushrooms
2 tsp paprika
flour to thicken
800ml stock
50ml white wine or sherry
1 tbsp Worcestershire sauce
140ml crème fraîche or sour cream
fresh parsley, chopped

Gently fry the onion, celery and garlic in a mix of butter and oil until soft. Add the mushrooms, then, when cooked, sprinkle with the paprika and a little flour, stir it around before adding the stock, wine or sherry and Worcestershire sauce. Bring to the boil, then simmer until it thickens. Stir in the crème fraîche or sour cream and gently heat through. Do not allow it to boil. Season to taste and serve with rice. Garnish with chopped parsley.

# BULGAR WHEAT WITH ROAST VEGETABLES

(3-4 SERVINGS)

### Roast Vegetables
1 red pepper, de-seeded
1 aubergine, cut into chunks
1 large onion, cut into wedges
1 large tomato
olive oil
balsamic vinegar

Cut the pepper into quarters. Put the vegetables into an oven-proof dish and drizzle generously with olive oil. Season, then toss the vegetables to coat them with the oil. Roast in a preheated oven at 180°C (gas mark 4) for 40–60 minutes. Turn the vegetables once or twice during this time and add a splash of balsamic vinegar near the end of the cooking period.

### Bulgar Wheat
1 clove garlic, peeled and cut thinly
4 tbsp olive oil or butter
120g bulgar wheat
chopped coriander/parsley
stock

Sweat the garlic in a saucepan in the oil or butter for 1 minute. Add the bulgar wheat and coriander and stir it around. Pour in enough stock to just cover the bulgar wheat, bring to the boil, then take off the heat and leave until the liquid is absorbed – about 10 minutes. Season, add any additions (peas, chopped red pepper etc.) and fluff up with a fork. Serve with the roast vegetables on top.

# FAVA – SPLIT-PEA MASH

## (4 SERVINGS)

*Traditionally part of a Greek meze, fava can be served with various toppings – capers, chopped tomatoes, cooked mushrooms, crisply fried onion, sausage or meatballs.*

180g split peas, green or yellow
3 cloves garlic, crushed
2 tbsp white wine
50ml olive oil
salt and freshly ground black pepper
2 tbsp white wine vinegar

Boil the split peas for 1 hour. Skim off any froth. Strain, then whizz in a processor with the garlic, wine and olive oil. Season to taste with salt, black pepper and wine vinegar. It should be thick.


# SPICY POTATO SKINS

## (6–8 SERVINGS)

*A whole baked potato has a very high GI but its skin contains fibre and potassium and has a high nutritional value.*

4 medium baking potatoes
$1/2$ tsp black pepper
1 heaped tsp curry powder
1 heaped tsp ground coriander

Cut the potatoes in half lengthways. Place them cut-side down on an oiled baking tray and bake in a preheated oven at 200°C (gas mark 6) for 30 minutes, or until soft. Run a pointed knife around the rim of each potato half, then scoop out the flesh leaving just a centimetre of flesh against the potato skin.

**Optional:** bake an onion in its skin as the potatoes cook, then remove the onion skin and mash the soft onion with flavouring to use as a filler.

*To serve as nibbles with drinks:* cut each potato skin into three wedges, then put the skins in a bowl, drizzle a little olive oil over and gently toss. Sprinkle the spice mixture over the skins. Bake at 160°C (gas mark 3) for 15 minutes until crisp and golden.

*To serve as a main meal:* put the potato halves into a bowl, drizzle a little olive oil over them, and gently toss. Sprinkle the spice mixture over the skins, then bake for 15 minutes until crisp and golden. Pile some filling into each half and serve with salad.

**Fillings**
Chilli bean mix or beans in marinara sauce (see page 121).

Tinned tuna (in oil) mashed with low-fat mayonnaise.

Anchovies chopped finely and mashed with baked onion, lemon juice and olive oil.

Ripe avocado mashed with Greek-style yoghurt, chopped tomato and a pinch of chilli.

Strips of smoked salmon mixed with Greek-style yoghurt, lemon juice and a few capers or chopped mini-gherkins.

# SWEET POTATOES

*These can be baked and served as chips or wedges,*
*or baked and stuffed with a savoury filling.*

**Chipped or wedged:** peel and cut potatoes into chunky chips or wedges. Tip into a bowl and spray with oil. Toss to make sure they have a covering. Spread on a baking tray, season and bake in a preheated oven at 180°C (gas mark 4) for 15 minutes. Turn the potatoes and bake for a further 15 minutes.

**Stuffed:** spray potatoes with oil and bake in a preheated oven at 160°C (gas mark 3) for about 30–40 minutes until soft. Scoop out the centres and mash with feta cheese, a generous dollop of mayonnaise, fresh chopped herbs and some butter or olive oil. Pile the filling back into the skins and serve with a green salad.

# Bean Mezze
# (with optional Meatballs or Chorizo)

(4 SERVINGS)

*This works equally well with combinations of green beans or a frozen mix of beans and peas. If the meat is omitted it can be served as a side dish.*

1 onion, chopped
2–4 cloves garlic, chopped
4 tbsp olive oil
1–2 tsp cumin
$\frac{1}{2}$ tsp chilli powder
1 tin chopped tomatoes
400g runner beans, chopped
400g frozen broad beans
50g fresh mint, chopped
extra olive oil
8 beef meatballs or 250g chorizo, cut into thick slices

Sweat the onion and garlic in oil until transparent. Add the cumin and chilli and cook for a few seconds. Empty the tinned tomatoes into the pan, then fill the empty tin with water and add that also. Stir in the beans and mint, then simmer until the liquid is reduced and thick. Stir in more oil to make the mezze thick and rich, and season to taste. Spoon the mezze into a baking dish, top with the meatballs or stir the chorizo into the mixture, and bake in a preheated oven at 160°C (gas mark 3) for 40 minutes until hot and bubbling.

# STUFFED PEPPERS GRATIN
## (with optional beef mince)

(4 SERVINGS)

*Minced beef can be used instead of mushrooms.*

100g sliced baby mushrooms (or mince)
50g breadcrumbs
2 cloves garlic, finely chopped
2 tbsp parsley, chopped
1 tsp paprika
2 tbsp tomato purée
1 onion, sliced very finely
2 large tomatoes, de-skinned and chopped
2 green peppers, halved and de-seeded
450ml thick cheese sauce (see page 100)
a little Parmesan, grated

Mix the mushrooms (or mince) with the breadcrumbs, garlic, parsley, paprika and tomato purée. (If using mushrooms sauté them first in a little butter.) Season. Spread the onion and tomatoes in an oven-proof dish and season well. Place the peppers in boiling water for 5–8 minutes until slightly softened. Drain and spoon the mixture into the pepper halves. Pat the mixture down firmly. Lay the peppers on top of the onion and tomatoes, then spoon a generous quantity of cheese sauce over this – make sure everything is covered. Sprinkle with Parmesan and bake in a preheated oven at 180°C (gas mark 4) for 30–40 minutes until the sauce is bubbling. Serve with a green vegetable.

# MAIN MEALS WITH RED MEAT

## SPICY LAMB CASSEROLE

(2 SERVINGS)

*A rich stew. Can be cooked in the oven or a slow cooker.*

1 tsp ground cardamom
1 tsp cinnamon
2 tbsp olive oil
200g lamb neck fillet, cut into pieces
4 baby onions, peeled
1 tbsp flour
a generous splash of red wine or port
200ml stock
3–4 dried prunes
fresh mint, chopped

Make a paste with the spices and oil, roll the lamb pieces in it, then gently fry in a little oil – brown the meat but do not let the spices burn. Remove the meat and add the onions (add a little extra oil if necessary). Cook for one minute, then return the meat to the pan. Stir in the flour, then add the wine or port, stock and prunes. Cook in a preheated oven at 150°C (gas mark 2) for 2 hours or in a slow cooker for 3–4 hours. Sprinkle with chopped mint and serve.

# LAMB TORTE

## (6-8 SERVINGS)

*This can be cooked a day ahead, then reheated. The meat is cooked in advance in a very slow oven. Adjust the quantity of beans and potatoes according to how many people are being served. One tin of beans will serve 2–3 people (to use dried beans see page 100). Do not peel the potatoes, and keep the large starchy potato for the top layer.*

shoulder of lamb, approx. 2.5kg
2 tbsp olive oil
6 cloves garlic, peeled and cut into slivers
150ml white wine
fresh rosemary, chopped
2 tins haricot beans, rinsed and drained
12 small potatoes, cut into small cubes
1 large onion, chopped
100g parsley, chopped
1 large potato

Trim off excess fat, then brown the meat in a little hot oil in a roasting tin. Cool slightly, then stab the meat and insert some of the garlic. Add the wine to a roasting tin with the rosemary. Cover the tin with foil, making sure the meat is totally sealed, and cook in a preheated oven at 120°C (gas mark ½) for 6 hours or longer – check and baste the meat occasionally during cooking.

When cooked, pull the meat off the bone, cover and put aside. Keep the meat juices (they will solidify and will need reheating if the torte is not being made immediately. The solid layer of fat can be taken off but some fat is needed to seal and then crisp the potato topping.)

*For the torte:* cover the base of a large baking dish with oil and garlic. Mix the remaining beans, potato cubes and onion together and cover the base of the dish with the mixture. Season and sprinkle with chopped rosemary and parsley. Layer the meat over the bean mixture to form a solid layer. Slice the large potato thinly and put overlapping slices on top. Season, then pour the meat juices over this. Make sure the top potato layer is coated — the fat in the meat juice will seal the potato and stop it discolouring. Cover and bake in a preheated oven at 160°C (gas mark 3) for approximately 1 hour depending upon the size of the torte. Leave uncovered near the end for the potato topping to go crisp and brown.

# LAMB CASSEROLE WITH CHICK-PEAS

(4 SERVINGS)

*Cook in the oven or a slow cooker.*

400g lamb neck fillet, cut into pieces
2 tbsp olive oil
1 large onion, sliced
3 cloves garlic, chopped fine
3 tomatoes, de-skinned and chopped
400g tin chick-peas
2 tsp ras el hanout (see page 101)
juice of 2 limes
4–6 dried apricots
100g spinach, chopped
fresh coriander, chopped

Brown the meat in hot oil for a minute or two, add the onion and garlic, cook on low until soft, then add everything else except the spinach and coriander. Cook in a preheated oven at 150°C (gas mark 2) for 2 hours or a slow cooker for 3–4 hours. The spinach and coriander should be stirred in a few minutes before the end of cooking time.

# MOROCCAN BEEF WITH LENTILS

## (2 SERVINGS)

*This dish can be cooked in a slow cooker for 3–4 hours.*
*Do not overcook as the lentils will not hold their shape.*

1 tsp cumin
2 tsp ras el hanout (see page 101)
1 garlic clove, crushed and sliced
100g frying steak, cut into strips
2 tbsp olive oil
1 onion, diced
50g lentils
small tin tomatoes, chopped
50g raisins
tomato ketchup
100–150ml stock
50g fresh mint or coriander

Mix the spices and garlic, then mix with the steak strips. Stir fry for a minute in hot oil, then put aside. Gently fry the onion until soft, then add the steak, lentils, tomatoes, raisins and some ketchup. Spoon into an oven-proof dish and add just enough stock to cover the mixture. Cover and bake in a preheated oven at 160°C (gas mark 3) for 1–1½ hours, giving an occasional stir through the cooking period. Garnish with chopped mint or coriander.

# PEPPERPOT BEEF

## (4 SERVINGS)

1 clove garlic, sliced
1 onion, sliced
2 tbsp oil
250g braising steak, diced
1 tin chopped tomatoes
½ tsp chilli powder
½ tsp ginger, fresh (grated) or ground
2 tbsp vinegar
freshly ground black pepper
120g button mushrooms, halved
1 tin baked beans

Gently fry the garlic and onion in te oil, then stir in and brown the meat. Mix the tomatoes with the spices, vinegar and freshly ground black pepper. Pour over the meat and onion. Cook in a preheated oven at 170ºC (between gas mark 3 and 4) for 2 hours. Add the mushrooms and beans 10 minutes before the end of cooking time.

# BEEF BARLEY STEW

## (4 SERVINGS)

*Barley stews are thick and warming and can be made in a slow cooker. Pearl barley increases in volume four- to six-fold when cooked, so a little goes a very long way.*

220g casserole beef, cubed
2 tbsp oil
1 large onion, chopped
2 cloves garlic, sliced
1 tin tomatoes, chopped
700ml stock or water
50g pearl barley
1 tbsp sweet paprika
sour cream to serve

Brown the meat in the oil. Add the onion and garlic and cook until the onion is soft. Stir in everything except the sour cream. Bring to a simmer, cover and cook until the barley and meat are tender – about 1 hour on the hob, 3–4 hours on high in a slow cooker. Serve in bowls with a swirl of sour cream.

# BEEF AND MUSHROOM BARLEY STEW

## (3–4 SERVINGS)

*As previously stated, pearl barley increases in volume four- to six-fold when cooked so a little goes a very long way. Cook on the hob or in a slow cooker.*

170g casserole beef, cubed
2 tbsp oil
1 large onion, chopped
170g large mushrooms, sliced
1 large carrot, sliced
40g pearl barley
500ml stock
250ml red wine
250ml tomato juice
120g frozen peas
1 tbsp lemon juice
sour cream to serve

Brown the meat in the oil. Add the onion and cook until soft. Stir in the mushrooms, carrot, barley, stock, wine and tomato juice. Bring to a simmer, then cover and cook until the meat and barley are tender – about 1 hour on the hob or 3–4 hours on high in a slow cooker. Add the peas and cook for 10 minutes, then add the lemon juice and season to taste. Serve in bowls with a swirl of sour cream.

# SAUSAGE AND MASH

## (2 SERVINGS)

*Mashing a vegetable in with potato will lower the GI of the potato. The GI will be reduced even further if the potato is allowed to cool and then reheated. In this recipe, potato is mashed with spinach. This is a variation of a Dutch recipe called* boerenkool. *In Holland the potato is mashed with kale and eaten with smoked sausage. To make it with kale, steam the kale over the boiling potatoes, then chop and mash with the cooked potato.*

2 medium potatoes
2 large onions, sliced
2 tbsp butter or oil
2–4 sausages with high meat content
butter and milk for mashing
100g fresh spinach, chopped

Peel and cut the potatoes into even sized chunks. Boil, then simmer until soft. Cook the onion slices gently in butter or oil until they are soft and caramelised. Grill or fry the sausages. When the sausages are cooked and brown put them on top of the fried onions and keep warm. Drain the potato, then mash with butter and a little milk. Season well. Stir the spinach into the potato and keep folding it in until the spinach is wilted. Divide the mash between two plates and pile the fried onion and sausages on top.

# SAUSAGE WITH LENTILS
### (4 SERVINGS)

300g Puy (black) lentils
2 onions, chopped
1 clove garlic, chopped
$\frac{1}{2}$ tsp ground cumin
a pinch of cayenne pepper
600ml stock
1 tbsp grain mustard
1 tsp lemon juice
2 tbsp oil
6 mushrooms
8 sausages with high meat content

Add the lentils, one of the onions, garlic, cumin and cayenne pepper to the stock, bring to the boil, then simmer for 35 minutes until the liquid is absorbed and the lentils are tender. Stir in the mustard, season and add the lemon juice. Fry the second onion in the oil. Fry or grill the mushrooms and the sausages, then cut into chunks. Mix in with the lentils and serve.

# ALTERNATIVES TO MASHED POTATO

*Dishes like fish and cottage pie are traditionally made with mashed potato but this has a high GI. Mashing a vegetable in with potato will lower its glycaemic impact. The GI will be reduced even further if the potato is allowed to cool and then reheated. Here are some alternative mashes. Cream, soy cream, olive oil or butter can all be used for mashing.*

## POTATO AND BEAN or CHICK-PEA MASH

(4 SERVINGS)

6 small – medium potatoes
tin cannellini beans or chick-peas, drained
1 large onion, chopped
2 tbsp oil or butter
1 tbsp cream
salt and freshly ground black pepper
Parmesan, grated

Boil the potatoes until soft. Strain and rinse the cannellini beans or chick-peas. Fry the onion in the oil or butter until transparent. Tip everything into a blender. Season well, then whizz up. Spread on top of a cottage pie mixture and top with some grated Parmesan. Bake in a preheated oven at 180°C (gas mark 4).

# CANNELLINI AND LEEK MASH

(4 SERVINGS)

1 large leek, cut into rings
1 clove garlic, chopped
2 tbsp oil or butter
tin cannellini beans, drained
salt and freshly ground black pepper
1 tbsp lemon juice
1 tbsp cream
Parmesan, grated

Gently cook the leek rings with the garlic in the oil or butter
until soft – 10–15 minutes. Stir the beans into the leeks, season
well, and mash with some lemon juice and cream. Spread on top
of a cottage pie mixture and top with grated Parmesan cheese.
Bake in a preheated oven at 180°C (gas mark 5).

# CAULIFLOWER MASH

## (4 SERVINGS)

*Cook and mash the cauliflower with a diced potato for more texture.*

1 cauliflower
1–2 tsp grain mustard
50ml single cream
salt and freshly ground black pepper
Parmesan, grated

Quarter a head of cauliflower, set aside the green bits and steam the rest until soft. Drain well, then mash with the mustard and single cream and season well. Sprinkle grated Parmesan over the top and grill or put in a preheated oven at 180°C (gas mark 5) for 20–30 minutes to brown.

## SWEET POTATO AND LEEK MASH

### (4 SERVINGS)

1 large sweet potato, peeled and cut into chunks
50ml plain yoghurt or single cream
1 large leek, cut into rings
1 tbsp butter
1–2 tsp grain mustard

Boil the sweet potato until soft. Drain, season and mash with the yoghurt or cream. Sweat the leek in the butter. When soft, mix in with the sweet potato. Add mustard, to taste.


## BROCCOLLI AND POTATO MASH

### (4 SERVINGS)

half a broccoli head
same volume of unpeeled potato, cut into chunks
crème fraîche or single cream
salt and freshly ground black pepper

Cut the broccoli into large florets and boil with the unpeeled potatoes. Drain, then mash with crème fraîche or single cream. Add a little milk if the mash is too thick. Season well.

# CHICKEN DISHES

## MOIST CHICKEN BREAST

*Chicken breasts can be dry, flavourless and disappointing.*
*This method of cooking keeps the meat moist.*

boneless chicken breasts, de-skinned
chopped mixed herbs, dried or fresh (optional)
flour
mix of olive oil and butter

Bash the chicken breasts with a rolling pin so that they are of an even thickness. Add the herbs to the flour, then toss the breasts in the flour. Heat the oil and butter in a pan. Turn the heat to medium and add the chicken breasts. Cook for 1 minute each side, then put a lid on the pan, turn the heat to its lowest level and leave it. *Do not lift the lid.* Cook for 8 minutes, giving the pan an occasional shake. When the 8 minutes are up, keep the pan covered (do not look), turn the heat off and leave the chicken in the covered pan for another 8 minutes. The breasts will be tender and ready for slicing.

# CHICKEN, CHORIZO AND BEANS

(4 SERVINGS)

*Cook on the hob or in a slow cooker.*

1 large onion, sliced
2 cloves garlic, chopped
2 tbsp olive oil
1 tin cannellini beans, rinsed and drained
4–6 chicken thighs, de-skinned
100g chorizo, thinly sliced
50g parsley, chopped
10 cherry tomatoes
400ml chicken stock
tomato paste

Sweat the onion and garlic in the oil until the onion is transparent. Keeping a few beans back, add the beans, chicken and chorizo to the pan. Cook gently for a few minutes. Whizz up the remaining beans (these will help to thicken the sauce), parsley and tomatoes in a blender and add to the pan. Season. Add the stock and tomato paste to taste, then the chicken and bean mixture. Simmer until the chicken is cooked.

# MOROCCAN CHICKEN AND LENTILS

## (2 SERVINGS)

*This dish can be cooked in a slow cooker on high for 3–4 hours (not for any longer, as the lentils will not hold their shape). The tomatoes can be fresh or tinned.*

1 tsp cumin
1 tsp crushed coriander seeds
1 tsp ras el hanout spice
1 clove garlic, crushed and sliced
2–4 chicken thighs, de-skinned
2 tbsp olive oil
tomatoes, de-skinned
1 onion, diced
50g lentils (any variety)
1 handful of raisins
Worcestershire or sweet chilli sauce
100–150ml stock
fresh coriander, chopped

Mix the spices and garlic, then mix with the chicken. Fry for 2 minutes in the oil, then put aside. Chop the tomatoes. Gently fry the onion until soft, then add the lentils, tomatoes, raisins and a splash of sauce. Stir in the chicken, then spoon into an oven-proof dish, add enough stock to cover the mixture, cover and bake in a preheated oven at 160°C (gas mark 3) for 1–1½ hours until the sauce is thick, stirring occasionally. Garnish with fresh coriander.

# CHICKEN WITH RED PEPPERS

## (4 SERVINGS)

*A recipe from northern Spain. Use sweet paprika for a mild dish or hot paprika for a spicier dish. This can also be made in a slow cooker.*

80g Serrano ham or thin slices of chorizo
1 onion, chopped
4 cloves garlic, chopped
2 tbsp olive oil
chicken pieces for 4, de-skinned
2 large red peppers, de-seeded and sliced
450g tomatoes, de-skinned and chopped
2 tsp paprika
a pinch of chilli
salt and freshly ground black pepper
50ml white wine (optional)
chopped parsley or coriander

Pull the ham into pieces. Sweat the onion and garlic in the oil, then add the chicken. Add the peppers and let them soften a little. Add the tomatoes to the pan with the ham and spices. Season, add the wine if using, cover and simmer for 1 hour (check and stir frequently to prevent sticking) or bake in a preheated oven at 180°C (gas mark 5). Remove the lid before the end of the cooking period to reduce the liquid. Serve with rice and garnish with chopped parsley or coriander.

# CHICKEN AND BROCCOLI CRUMBLE

## (4 SERVINGS)

8 chicken thighs, de-skinned
1 medium head of broccoli
300g condensed chicken or mushroom soup
2 tbsp low-fat mayonnaise
200ml crème fraîche
2 tsp lemon juice
120g wholemeal breadcrumbs
50g cheese grated

Cut the chicken and broccoli into bite-sized pieces and spread over the base of an oven-proof dish. Mix together the soup, mayonnaise, crème fraîche and lemon juice. Spoon over the chicken and broccoli. Mix together the breadcrumbs and cheese and cover the mixture. Bake in a preheated oven at 170°C (between gas mark 3 and 4) for 40–50 minutes.

# CURRIES AND ACCOMPANIMENTS

*Research indicates that some of the spices found in curry powders and pastes have health benefits. The GI of a curry meal will be significantly reduced if converted rice is used.*

## BASIC LOW-GI CURRY SAUCE
(3–4 SERVINGS)

*Use as the base for any combination of meat and vegetables.*

500ml stock
1 tsp cumin
1 tsp chilli or curry powder
1 tsp ginger, fresh, peeled and chopped or dried
1 tsp turmeric
1 tsp ground cardamom
1 tsp cinnamon
2 tsp ground coriander
2 onions, diced
2 cloves garlic, chopped
2 tbsp oil or melted butter
1 carrot, grated
fresh coriander and/or parsley, chopped

Pour the stock into a saucepan, put in all the spices and boil until reduced by half. Sweat the onions and garlic in the oil or butter until the onion is soft. Add the carrot, cook for another minute, then add the chopped herbs. Put this and the reduced stock into a blender and whizz. It should now have the consistency of a curry sauce – if too thin, continue cooking until it is thick enough.

# BASIC SAVOURY RICE

(2–3 SERVINGS)

50g button mushrooms, sliced
2 tbsp melted butter or oil
1 large leek, chopped
2 tsp curry powder or 1 tsp curry paste
200g cooked rice, basmati or converted

Cook the mushrooms in the melted butter, then set aside. Add more butter or oil and stir in the leek. Cover and cook on a very low heat until soft. Stir the curry powder or paste into the leek, then mix in the rice and mushrooms. Heat through and serve.


# FRIED RICE WITH EGG

(2–3 SERVINGS)

cooked basic savoury rice
1 tbsp oil or melted butter
2 eggs

Follow the recipe for basic savoury rice using a frying pan and push the rice/leek mixture around the edge of the pan. Pour the melted butter or oil into the centre of the pan, then break the eggs into the centre and scramble them. When just cooked stir the egg into the rice mixture.

# HERBY RICE AND LENTILS

## (4 SERVINGS)

*Mixing lentils with rice reduces the glycaemic impact of rice. It can be prepared in advance and heated through when required.*

125g green lentils
1 onion, chopped finely
2 tbsp oil or melted butter
big handful of fresh parsley and/or coriander
500g cooked rice, basmati or converted
butter

Cook the lentils in boiling water for about 10 minutes, until tender, then drain and leave until dry. Gently cook the onion in the oil or butter until soft and slightly browned at the edges. Chop the herbs. Mix everything together, pile into an oven-proof dish, dot with butter, cover and heat through in a preheated oven at 150°C (gas mark 2) or microwave.

# LENTIL AND SPINACH CURRY

(4–6 SERVINGS)

*A very aromatic curry.*

110g Puy (black) lentils
300ml chicken or vegetable stock
2 tbsp oil
2 large onions, sliced
1 tsp ground cumin
1 tbsp ground coriander
½ tsp curry or chilli powder
100g baby spinach leaves
fresh coriander

Put the lentils in a heavy-based saucepan and cover generously with the stock. Bring to the boil, then simmer for 30 minutes, stirring regularly. Heat the oil in a large frying pan. Add the onions and spices and stir around so the onion is well coated – top up the oil if necessary. Cover and cook until soft and browned in places. Fold in the spinach – this will take 2–3 minutes and is best done handful by handful. When the spinach is wilted, add the cooked lentils. Heat through, serve with basmati or converted rice and garnish with chopped coriander.

# SPINACH, LENTIL AND POTATO CURRY

## (4 SERVINGS)

2 cloves garlic, chopped
2 tsp medium hot curry paste
1 tsp cumin powder
1 tsp turmeric
2 tbsp oil
6 small potatoes, unpeeled and quartered
100g red lentils
2 tomatoes, chopped
2 carrots, chopped
a large bunch of parsley, chopped
300ml stock
1 bag spinach

Gently fry the garlic and spices in the oil for 2 minutes. Add the potatoes, lentils, tomatoes, carrots and parsley. Cover generously with the stock, bring to the boil, then reduce to a simmer. Add the spinach a handful at a time and stir it in until it wilts. Simmer for 30–40 minutes until the vegetables and lentils are cooked, or in a slow cooker on low, where it can be left until required. Serve with basmati or converted rice.

# QUICK VEGETABLE CURRY

## (2 SERVINGS)

*Any left-over vegetable can be used up in this curry but tomatoes
or a sliced red pepper give the necessary moisture.
Some jalapeno pepper will add zing.*

1 onion, chopped small
1 clove garlic, chopped
fresh ginger, grated
2 tbsp oil or melted butter
1 tsp Thai curry paste
½ aubergine, sliced then diced
2 large tomatoes, chopped
2 small potatoes, diced
2 carrots, diced
5 tbsp water or stock

Sweat the onion with the garlic and ginger in the oil or butter
until the onion is transparent. Stir in the curry paste. Add the
aubergine and cook for another few minutes, then add everything
else. Top up with water or stock, cover and cook on a very low
heat – add more water or stock if the curry dries out too much.
Serve with basmati or converted rice.

# CHICKEN CURRY IN COCONUT MILK

## (2 SERVINGS)

*A curry quickly made with a diced chicken breast or thigh.
Add peas, chopped red pepper, sweetcorn etc. to taste.*

200g uncooked chicken pieces
1 onion, chopped
1 clove garlic, crushed and chopped
a knob of fresh ginger, grated
2 tbsp oil or melted butter
1 tbsp Thai curry paste
800ml stock
50g creamed coconut, cut into small pieces
chopped coriander

De-skin the chicken. Sweat the onion, garlic and ginger in the oil or butter until the onion is transparent, then stir in the curry paste and chicken pieces. Stir around and cook for a few minutes. Add the stock and coconut cream. Simmer and stir until the coconut is dissolved, then continue simmering until the chicken is cooked. Serve with basmati or converted rice and garnish with coriander.

# PRAWN LAKSA

## (4 SERVINGS)

*A spicy noodle soup with a coconut curry base.*

200g uncooked noodles
1–2 tbsp green Thai curry paste
400ml coconut milk
400ml vegetable or chicken stock
1 red pepper, de-seeded and chopped
50g mange-tout peas
50g spinach
8–12 cooked prawns
coriander, chopped
2 spring onions, cut on the slant

Pour boiling water over the noodles and set aside for 5 minutes, stirring occasionally to prevent them sticking. Put the curry paste in a wok or deep saucepan, add some coconut milk and stir into a thick sauce. Simmer for 2 minutes, then add the remaining coconut milk and the stock and simmer for another minute. Just before serving, add the red pepper and mange-touts and simmer for a few minutes. Then add the spinach and stir until wilted. Add the drained noodles and prawns, heat through, then serve in bowls, garnished with chopped coriander and spring onions.

# LASSI

Lassi is the drink that takes the heat out of a curry. It is made with one part natural yoghurt to three parts water. Traditionally, freshly ground black pepper and salt are added with chopped mint or coriander leaves. The mix is left to stand to allow the flavours to develop, then served chilled. A sweet lassi is made by mixing the yoghurt and water with mango purée, leaving out the salt and pepper and adding sweetener, to taste.

# LOW-SUGAR CHUTNEY

*Make this with plum, apricot or mango. It will fill one large jam-jar.*

small piece of root ginger
330g fresh fruit, weight de-stoned
1 red onion, chopped finely
50ml red wine vinegar
70g raisins
1 tsp cinnamon
½ tsp chilli (optional)
115ml prune or orange juice
20g brown sugar

Peel and finely chop the ginger. Chop the fruit. Put everything into a large shallow pan, bring to the boil, then simmer for 30 minutes until the onion is soft and the chutney is thick (it will thicken further as it cools). Stir frequently to prevent catching. Store in the fridge when cool.

# YOGHURT AND MINT RELISH

A cooling side dish to go with curry.

4 tbsp natural yoghurt
1 tbsp fresh mint, chopped finely
$\frac{1}{2}$ tsp chilli powder
$\frac{1}{2}$ tsp salt

First whisk the yoghurt, then whisk in everything else. Serve slightly chilled.

# SEAFOOD AND SAUCES

## FISHCAKES
### (MAKES 4–5 FISHCAKES)

300g any white fish
milk to cover the fish
2 medium potatoes
1 tbsp tartare sauce, English style (see page 171)
zest from 1 lemon
parsley, chopped
spring onion, finely chopped
oat flakes, if frying
1 egg, beaten, for frying method

Poach the fish in the milk – bring to the boil, simmer for 4 minutes, then take off the heat and stand for 10 minutes. Drain the fish. Dice then boil the potato until soft, then drain and allow to dry. Mash with a fork, season well and stir in the tartare sauce, then add the fish, lemon zest, parsley and onion. Divide into 4 or 5 fishcakes. They can now be grilled, baked or fried.

**To grill or bake:** brush with olive oil and grill or bake at 160°C (gas mark 3) until nicely browned.

**To fry:** whizz up some oat flakes in a food processor to make oatmeal. Roll each fishcake in beaten egg and then in the oatmeal. Fry in hot oil.

# SALMON WITH BEAN MASH

(2–3 SERVINGS)

2 cloves garlic, chopped
1 tsp ground cumin
1 tbsp olive oil
zest and juice of 1 lemon
400g tin cannellini beans, rinsed and drained
2–3 anchovies
200g salmon
parsley, chopped
1 tsp capers, rinsed and drained
1 spring onion, chopped

Gently cook the garlic and cumin in the oil. Retain some lemon juice for the dressing – add the rest plus the zest to the garlic, cook for 2 minutes, then add the beans. Tip the bean mixture and anchovies into a blender and whizz together – it does not need to be smooth. Keep warm. Cook the salmon (poach or microwave), de-skin and break the fish into flakes. Mix the parsley, capers and spring onion together, then mix with the remaining lemon juice and a little oil. Serve the salmon on top of the mash and spoon the parsley-lemon mixture over the salmon.

# CRAB PASTA
## (2 SERVINGS)

1 clove garlic, chopped
1 onion, chopped very small
1 tbsp oil or melted butter
150ml chicken stock
1 tsp tomato paste
1 dressed crab, medium
150ml single cream
a pinch of cayenne pepper
200g cooked spaghetti
fresh parsley, chopped

Sweat the garlic and onion in the oil or butter until soft. Add the stock, tomato paste and all the crab meat (white and brown). Simmer gently for 5 minutes, then stir in the cream. Add the pepper and heat through but do not allow to boil. Stir in the spaghetti, heat through and serve garnished with parsley.

# CRAB CAKES

(MAKES 8 SMALL CAKES)

1 medium potato
1 dressed crab, medium
2 spring onions, finely chopped
1 tsp capers, chopped finely
1 tbsp mayonnaise
1 tbsp lemon juice
a pinch of chilli
oat flakes, if frying
1 egg, beaten, for frying method

Cook the potato then drain and leave for a few moments to dry. Mash, stir in the crab meat (white and brown), spring onions, capers, mayonnaise, lemon juice and chilli, season, then shape into 8 small round patties. Put aside in the fridge for 30 minutes – this will help them keep their shape when being cooked.

**To grill or bake:** brush with olive oil and grill or bake at 160°C (gas mark 3) until nicely browned.

**To fry:** whizz up some oat flakes in a food processor to make oatmeal. Roll each crab cake in beaten egg and then in the oatmeal. Fry in hot oil.

# MACKEREL FILLETS

*Mackerel is a strongly flavoured oily fish. The fishmonger will gut it if asked. Before cooking wash the fish under cold water and pat dry. Grilled mackerel needs the contrast of something sharp – traditionally rhubarb or gooseberry sauce. WARNING: strong cooking smells! To avoid this, wrap the fish in foil and cook in the oven or steam.*

**To fillet a mackerel:** cut off the head and tail. Extend the fishmonger's cut along the belly, then open the fish out like a book and lay the flesh side down on a board. Bash the length of the spine with a rolling pin, then turn the fish over and gently pull out the spine – all the little bones should come with it. Trim the edges of any spiny bits.

# MACKEREL IN OATMEAL
(2 SERVINGS)

*Whizz up oat flakes in a food processer to make oatmeal.
This is traditionally eaten with mayonnaise flavoured
with grain or Dijon mustard.*

2 mackerel fillets
oatmeal
oil, for frying
lemon wedges, to serve

Roll the fillets in well-seasoned oatmeal, pressing the oatmeal on
and covering them generously. Heat some oil in a frying pan, and
gently fry the fillets until golden brown – about 2 minutes each
side. Serve with lemon wedges.


# BAKED MACKEREL FILLETS
# WITH CORIANDER AND LEMON
(2 SERVINGS)

4 small mackerel fillets
2 tbsp fresh coriander, chopped
1 tbsp lemon juice

Lay the fillets in a baking dish and cover with the coriander.
Sprinkle with the lemon juice and bake in a preheated oven at
180°C (gas mark 5) for 5–10 minutes each side or microwave for
2 minutes.

# BAKED MACKEREL FILLETS
# WITH PAPRIKA AND LEMON
(2 SERVINGS)

½ tsp paprika
1 tbsp lemon juice
4 small mackerel fillets

Make a paste with the paprika and lemon juice. Roll the mackerel fillets in the paste, then bake in a preheated oven at 160°C (gas mark 3) for 5–10 minutes or microwave for 2 minutes.

# GOOSEBERRY SAUCE
(2 SERVINGS)

100g gooseberries
20g melted butter
2 tbsp cream
sweetener, to taste
salt and pepper

Top and tail the gooseberries. Chop, then sweat them in the butter until soft. Mash them, then stir in the cream, salt and freshly ground black pepper. Add sweetener.

# RHUBARB SAUCE

## (2 SERVINGS)

*This sauce also goes well with salmon and pork.*

1 tsp fresh ginger, grated
20g melted butter
2 sticks of rhubarb, cut into pieces
a pinch of grated nutmeg
chopped sorrel
sweetener, to taste

Gently sweat the fresh ginger in the butter. Stew the rhubarb with a little water until soft. Add the butter, ginger and nutmeg, simmer for 10 minutes, then add the sorrel and sweetener, to taste. Whizz in a blender until smooth.

# MACKEREL ON PESTO MASH

(2 SERVINGS)

1 large mackerel fillet
1 medium potato, cut into chunks
1 onion, chopped small
1–2 tbsp fresh pesto
olive oil
1 large tomato, sliced
breadcrumbs, whizzed up fine

Trim the edge of the mackerel of any spiny bits. Boil then drain the potato. Tip into a blender with the onion and pesto. Whizz until smooth. Spoon the mash into an oven-proof dish and lay the fish on top, flesh side down. Brush the mackerel skin with olive oil and surround it with slices of tomato. Season well, scatter with breadcrumbs and drizzle with a little olive oil. Bake in a preheated oven at 180°C (gas mark 4) for 20–25 minutes. Cut the fillet in half and serve.

# TARTARE SAUCE ENGLISH STYLE

(4–6 SERVINGS)

3 tbsp low-fat mayonnaise
1 tsp cream of horseradish
1 tsp grain mustard
squeeze of lemon juice
1 tbsp capers, drained and chopped
2 tsp onion, chopped finely
1 tbsp mini-gherkins, drained and chopped
fresh parsley, chopped finely

Whisk everything together and allow to stand for 1 hour before serving.

# TARTARE SAUCE AMERICAN STYLE

(4–6 SERVINGS)

3 tbsp low-fat mayonnaise
1 tsp sweet pickle
2 tsp onion, chopped finely
1 tsp lemon juice
salt and black pepper, to taste

Whisk everything together and allow to stand for 1 hour before serving.


# HERBY MAYONNAISE

(4–6 SERVINGS)

3 tbsp low-fat mayonnaise
chopped dill or parsley
1 egg, beaten
1 tbsp lemon juice
4 tbsp Greek yoghurt

Mix the mayonnaise, dill or parsley and egg. Add the lemon juice and any fish juices. Heat gently until the mixture thickens – do not allow the mixture to boil. Stir the yoghurt into the mixture.

# HERBY SAUCE FOR POACHED SALMON
### (4–6 SERVINGS)

*A recipe adapted from one seen on television.*

equal measure of vinegar and olive oil
1 onion, chopped very small
2 tsp tomato ketchup
1 tsp Worcestershire sauce
5 drops of Tabasco
lots of fresh herbs, chopped finely

Whisk everything together – the sauce should be thick and green.
Season and spoon over cooked salmon.

# SALADS

## SALAD DRESSING

*Use an equal amount of vinegar and oil and whisk everything together.*

1 clove garlic, crushed then sliced
50ml sherry or cider vinegar
dash of Worcestershire sauce
50ml olive oil
salt and pepper, to taste
sweetener, to taste
fresh thyme leaves (optional)

## DIJON BUTTERMILK DRESSING

*This goes well with seafood. Whisk everything together.*

300ml buttermilk
1 tbsp Dijon mustard
1 tbsp cider vinegar
sweetener, to taste

# NICOISE SALAD WITH FISHCAKE

(2 SERVINGS)

1–2 hard-boiled eggs
2–3 small potatoes, cooked and sliced
1 pack French green beans, cooked
50g black olives, de-stoned
cherry tomatoes, halved
salad leaves
salad dressing
1–2 fishcakes
spring onions, cut on the slant

Cut the eggs into quarters. Gently mix the potatoes, beans, olives, tomatoes and salad leaves. Toss in the dressing, then add the egg quarters. Cook the fishcakes (see page 163), slice them and serve on top of the salad.

# LEMON AND BUTTER BEAN SALAD

(4 SERVINGS)

*A substantial salad that goes well with cold meat or fish.*
*Add a small tin of tuna to turn it into a complete meal.*

spring onions
1 pack of asparagus or French beans
2 cloves garlic, peeled and crushed
sea salt
zest and juice of 1 lemon
parsley, chopped finely
1 tbsp olive oil
1 tin butter beans, drained and rinsed
50g frozen peas
3–4 small potatoes, cooked and sliced

Cut the spring onions into shortish lengths. Steam the asparagus or beans until just tender, then drain and cut these too into shortish lengths. Make a dressing for the salad by pounding the crushed garlic with some crunchy sea salt in a pestle and mortar, then adding the lemon zest and juice and chopped parsley. Tip this into a largish bowl and add the olive oil. Season to taste. Mix everything together and serve at room temperature.

# TUNA AND BEAN SALAD

## (2 SERVINGS)

*A classic Italian salad. Make it an hour or two in advance to allow the flavours to blend.*

half tin cannellini beans
small tin tuna (in oil)
1 clove garlic, chopped finely
1 tbsp balsamic vinegar
1 tbsp olive oil
1 spring onion, sliced
cherry tomatoes, halved
handful of basil leaves, chopped

Drain and rinse the beans and the tuna. Combine the garlic, vinegar and olive oil to make a dressing. Toss everything else together, then drizzle the dressing over the salad.

# RICE SALAD WITH SMOKED MACKEREL

## (4 SERVINGS)

*The feta will crumble more easily if put in the freezer for a few minutes before using.*

120g basmati or converted rice
2 peppered mackerel fillets
2 dried apricots, sliced
watercress, torn into shreds
cherry tomatoes, halved
1 spring onion, sliced
50g sunflower seeds
70g crumbled feta
a few almonds (optional)

Cook the rice. De-skin the mackerel, then flake the fish and discard the skin. If possible, toss the rice and fish together while the rice is still hot. Cool, then toss everything else in and let the salad stand for 10 minutes or more before serving.

# FILLET OF BEEF SALAD

(2 SERVINGS)

1 piece of beef fillet
red wine to cover beef
green salad
new potatoes in savoury dressing (see page 180)

Cut the beef fillet into 1cm slices with a very sharp knife. Marinate in red wine for up to 24 hours in the fridge, turning occasionally. Stretch each piece of beef to extend it. Cook on a hot griddle for 90 seconds each side. Serve with its juices over a green salad and with new potatoes in a savoury dressing.

# NEW POTATOES IN SAVOURY DRESSING

(3–4 SERVINGS)

2 tbsp grain mustard
1 tbsp red wine vinegar
6 tbsp extra-virgin olive oil
3–4 small new potatoes, cooked and sliced
chopped parsley
2 tbsp capers
sliced gherkins

Whisk the mustard and vinegar together, then add the oil bit by bit. It will go thick. Stir it into the potatoes, parsley and pickles.

# GREEK SALAD

## (2–3 SERVINGS)

4 tomatoes
sea salt
a pinch of sugar
half a cucumber
1 small red onion
herby black olives
lemon juice
olive oil
freshly ground black pepper
fresh coriander/mint/parsley
feta cheese

De-core the tomatoes, then cut them into wedges. Sprinkle with the salt and sugar. Cut the cucumber into wedges. Slice the onion thinly. Gently mix the tomatoes, onion, cucumber and olives together. Make a dressing with lemon juice, olive oil and pepper. Pour over the salad. Just before serving, chop the herbs and mix in with the salad. Serve with slices of feta on top.

# RUSSIAN SALAD

## (6 SERVINGS)

*The flavour improves if made a day in advance.*

6 small waxy potatoes, cooked
2 medium carrots, cooked and diced
50g peas, frozen
1 red pepper, de-skinned, de-seeded and diced
1 small tin tuna (in oil)
2 tbsp mayonnaise
green olives, chopped
2 hard-boiled eggs (optional)

De-skin the potatoes when cool enough, then dice. Mix the vegetables and tuna together, including the oil. Season well, fold in the mayonnaise and olives, then chill for at least 1 hour, preferably longer. To serve, pile the salad into a mound in the centre of a plate and surround it with slices of hard-boiled egg.

# CHICK-PEA SALAD

(4 SERVINGS)

1 tin chick-peas, drained
spring onions, chopped
radishes, sliced
romaine lettuce, chopped
baby tomatoes, halved
red and/or green pepper, de-seeded and chopped
100g Edam cheese, cubed
50g salami or pastrami, cut into strips
salad dressing (see page 174)

Combine the chick-peas with the vegetables, cheese and salami or pastrami strips. Make the dressing and pour over the mixture. Leave to stand for 30 minutes. Stir before serving.

*Chick-pea salad for a party:* use dried chick-peas. Allow 60g of dried chick-peas per person and soak the peas overnight. Bring to the boil in fresh water, then simmer for 30–40 minutes until soft.

# WATERCRESS AND MINT SALAD

## (4 SERVINGS)

*This is a nice winter salad although small courgettes can be hard to find.*

2 baby courgettes, sliced diagonally
pack of French green beans
50g frozen peas, defrosted
6 radishes, sliced into quarters lengthways
salad dressing
pack of watercress or rocket
50g mint leaves, chopped

Steam the courgettes and beans for 3–4 minutes only. Mix the non-leafy vegetables together and toss in a dressing. Add the watercress and mint leaves just before serving.

# PUDDINGS–JUST A FEW

*In all of these recipes sugar can be replaced with Truvia Baking Blend. This is twice as sweet as sugar so just halve the weight of sugar and replace it with the Truvia. For example, if a recipe calls for 100g sugar, use 50g Truvia.*

## SPICED HONEY ORANGES WITH YOGHURT
### (4 SERVINGS)

3 oranges
½ tsp ground cardamom
4 cloves, crushed
3 tsp honey
1 tsp vanilla essence
low-fat Greek yoghurt

Squeeze the juice from two of the oranges. Add the spices, honey and vanilla to the juice, bring to the boil, then cook until reduced by about half. Remove the peel and pith from the third orange and cut into very thin slices. Pour the syrup over the orange slices. Cool and serve with yoghurt.

# SCOTTISH CRANACHAN
## (2 SERVINGS)

*Whizz up some oat flakes in a food processor to make oatmeal.*

1 tbsp oatmeal
2 tbsp liquid honey mixed with 1 tbsp whisky
140ml double cream, whipped
100g fresh raspberries
1–2 tsp sugar or sweetener

Toast the oatmeal, then cool it. Fold the honey mixture into the cream. Mash the raspberries with a little sugar or sweetener. Gently mix everything together.

# BASMATI RICE PUDDING

(4 SERVINGS)

750ml milk
120g basmati rice
sweetener
1 tsp vanilla essence
½ tsp ground cardamom/cinnamon
single cream
a mix of fresh berries – raspberries, red currants etc.

Use a heavy saucepan to bring the milk and rice to the boil, then simmer for about 30 minutes, stirring now and then, until the rice is cooked. Add sweetener to taste, and the vanilla and spice. Spoon into individual dishes and serve hot or cold with a swirl of single cream and berries on top.

# LITTLE POTS OF CHOCOLATE

(4 SERVINGS)

*These should be made in little pots or dessert coffee cups,*
*as the mousse is thick, rich and smooth.*

150–200g plain chocolate
284ml single cream
2 egg yolks
20g soft butter
2 tbsp brandy (optional)

Break the chocolate into small pieces. Heat the cream until it is just about to boil, then take it off the heat. Drop the chocolate into the cream and stir it until melted. Stir in the yolks, butter and brandy. Spoon into little receptacles and chill for 2–3 hours before serving.

# MANGO FOOL
## (2–4 SERVINGS)

280ml double cream
fresh mango, peeled and diced
juice of 1 lime

Whisk the double cream until thick. Add some diced mango and lime juice and whisk again. Serve chilled.


# FRESH MANGO WITH SPICY SYRUP
## (3–4 SERVINGS)

juice from 1 lime
4 tbsp water
1 tsp sugar
$\frac{1}{2}$ tsp ground cardamom
chopped mint
1 mango, peeled and cut into slices

Combine the lime juice, water, sugar and cardamom and boil in a small saucepan until reduced by half. Add the mint and leave to cool. Put the mango slices into individual dishes and pour the strained syrup over.

# CAKES AND BISCUITS

*In all of these recipes, sugar can be replaced with Truvia Baking Blend. This is twice as sweet as sugar so just halve the weight of sugar and replace it with the Truvia. For example, if a recipe calls for 100g of sugar, use 50g of Truvia.*

## OATY BARS

(MAKES 20 SMALL SQUARES)

*Add extra bits – raisins, chopped apricots, chopped nuts, chocolate drops, chopped stem ginger etc. A large saucepan or wok is needed to mix the ingredients. The ratio of oat flakes to flour can be altered – the more oat flakes, the more crumbly the biscuit.*

160g butter
2 tbsp peanut butter
70g brown sugar
2 tbsp agave or honey
180g wholemeal or spelt flour
180g oat flakes
2 tsp cinnamon or mixed spice

Melt the butter in a large pan with the peanut butter, sugar and agave or honey. Stir in everything else, mix well, then spoon into a rectangular or square baking tray. Spread the mixture evenly over the base and pat down to make it firm. Bake in a preheated oven at 180°C (gas mark 4) for around 20 minutes, until the top is lightly browned. Leave to cool in the tin for 5 minutes, then score into square or finger shapes. Leave to cool and harden in the baking tray before turning out.

# SPICED HONEY AND RYE CAKE

### (MAKE IN A 17CM LOAF TIN)

2 tbsp honey
1 tbsp black treacle
80g brown sugar
$1/2$ tsp each of ground cloves, cinnamon, mace and ginger
$1/2$ tsp black pepper
150g butter, cubed
3 eggs
zest and pulp of 1 orange
50g mixed fruit
200g rye flour
$3/4$ tsp baking powder

Warm the honey, treacle, sugar and spices in a large pan until almost simmering. Remove from the heat and stir in the butter and let it melt. Beat the eggs into the mixture with the orange zest and pulp, mixed fruit, flour and baking powder. Spoon into a greased tin and bake in a preheated oven at 180°C (gas mark 4) for 50–60 minutes.

# OATMEAL BROONIE CAKE
### (MAKE IN A 17CM LOAF TIN)

*Broonie is a traditional Orkney gingerbread.*
*The treacle can be replaced with another sweetener*
*but the traditional taste of broonie will then be lost.*

170g wholemeal flour
½ tsp bicarb of soda
2–3 tsp ground ginger
170g medium oatmeal
60g soft brown sugar
90g butter
2 tbsp black treacle or syrup
280ml buttermilk or yoghurt
1 egg, beaten
50g sultanas or raisins
crystallised or stem ginger, chopped (optional)

Mix the dry ingredients together. Melt the butter and treacle or syrup in a pan, add the buttermilk or yoghurt and the beaten egg. Pour the liquid mixture into the dry ingredients and mix well. Stir in the sultanas or raisins. Spoon the mixture into a greased loaf tin and bake in a preheated oven at 180°C (gas mark 4). for 45–50 minutes until just firm in the middle.

# WHISKY BROONIE

Cover the sultanas or raisins with whisky and leave to soak for 2–3 hours or overnight. Follow the recipe for broonie but replace some of the buttermilk with the whisky used to soak the fruit.

# SWEDISH APPLE CAKE

(MAKE IN A 20CM SQUARE CAKE TIN)

*This cake uses white flour — for an occasional treat only.*

1 tbsp sugar
50g flaked almonds
85g butter
140g sugar
2 eggs
6 tbsp milk
230g self-raising white flour
3–4 large tart apples, de-cored and cubed
extra sugar for base of cake

Generously sprinkle the base of the cake tin with the sugar and the flaked almonds. Cream the butter and sugar together, add the eggs and milk, sieve in the flour, then fold in the apple cubes. Mix well and tip into the greased cake tin. Bake in a preheated oven at 180°C (gas mark 4) for 30–40 minutes. Leave to cool in the tin, then turn the cake out and serve upside down.

# NO-FLOUR CHOCOLATE BROWNIES

250g chocolate, mix of plain and dark
400g tin chick-peas, drained and rinsed
4 eggs
150g sugar
½ tsp baking powder
1 tsp vanilla essence
some broken nuts

Melt the chocolate in a bowl over boiling water. Blend the chick-peas, eggs, sugar and baking powder in a food processor until smooth. Transfer into a large bowl and pour in the melted chocolate. Add the vanilla then mix until smooth. Add the nuts, then pour the mixture into a greased loaf tin and bake in a preheated oven at 180°C (gas mark 4) for 30–40 minutes. Leave to cool in the tin before turning out.

# PASTRY

*Pastry made with wholemeal flour, rye or spelt flour should have a lower GI than pastry made with white flour. The ratio of wholemeal to white flour can be altered and rye or spelt flour used in the first two recipes. These make enough pastry to line two medium-sized flan cases.*

## PASTRY with vegetable oil

100g wholemeal flour
100g white flour
½ tsp salt
50ml vegetable oil
50ml water

Mix everything in a food processor. Add more flour or water if the consistency is too liquid or too stiff. Turn onto a board and mould into a dough. Wrap the dough in a plastic bag and leave in the fridge for 20–30 minutes before using.

# PASTRY with butter

100g wholemeal or spelt flour
100g white flour
90g butter, diced
a pinch of salt
1 egg yolk
50ml water

Whizz the flours with the butter and salt in a food processor. Add the egg yolk and just enough water to make a non-sticky dough. Turn onto a board and mould. Wrap the dough in a plastic bag and keep in the fridge for 20–30 minutes before using.

# MULTIGRAIN BREADMAKER LOAF

## (MAKES 1 SMALL LOAF)

*The addition of some strong white flour lightens the texture of the loaf. Best results are with strong Canadian white flour. The ratio and types of flour can be varied so long as there is a total quantity of 480g.*

160g strong wholemeal flour
130g strong white flour
160g rye flour
30g bran
325ml water
1 tsp dry yeast or one 7g packet
2 tsp vegetable oil
1 tsp salt
1 tsp sugar
seeds, chopped nuts etc. (optional)

Put everything into the bread machine and cook on the 3-hour setting.

# COOKING WITH COCONUT FLOUR

Coconut flour is very dry and needs a lot of liquid – recipes using coconut flour use a surprisingly small amount of coconut flour and a large amount of water and eggs. Coconut flour pastry does not roll out well – it crumbles and breaks. It is better to squash the dough, or break off lumps, and press it into the pie or flan tin. The pastry, when baked, tastes faintly of coconut, is slightly sweet and will not be to everyone's taste.

A mixture of spelt or wheat with coconut flour may be preferable but do not try to make straight swaps when adapting recipes. **As a general principle, remove a whole cupful of wheat flour and replace it with a third of a cup of coconut flour, an egg and a little extra water.** Coconut flour is expensive but a little goes a long way. It absorbs moisture very readily so must be kept in an airtight bag in a dry atmosphere – not in the fridge.

*Cooking with Coconut Flour* by Bruce Fife explains the principles of cooking with coconut flour and gives gluten-free recipes for a whole range of baked goods. Some of the recipes are high on sugar but this can be replaced with a sweetener.

# COCONUT FLOUR PASTRY

### (ENOUGH FOR 10 SMALL MINCE PIES)

70g coconut flour
100g butter, cut into lumps
a pinch of salt
1 egg
60g water

Whizz up the flour, butter and salt in a food processor until the mix looks like breadcrumbs. Add the egg and water. Whizz again, then turn out onto a board and knead to form a dough. Cover and leave in the fridge for 15 minutes or longer. When used, the dough will be unlike conventional pastry dough. Rolling it out will be almost impossible – instead, press lumps to line the baking container thinly. Bake in a preheated oven at 180°C (gas mark 4) for 15–20 minutes, until firm and slightly golden. **Leave the cooked pastry to cool in its bun tin;** otherwise it will crumble and collapse.

# SPELT AND COCONUT FLOUR PASTRY

120g spelt or wholemeal flour
30g coconut flour
cup of water and vegetable oil, mixed
1 egg

Whizz everything up in a food processor, then turn out the dough onto a board and knead. It will be quite moist. Cover and leave in the fridge for 15 minutes or longer. Sprinkle the dough and worktop with flour before rolling out. Use for pies, flans, sausage rolls etc.

# PANCAKES with coconut flour

## (MAKES 10–12 SMALL PANCAKES)

*These are best made in a small frying pan, diameter 16cm.*
*The pancakes tend to break up when made in a bigger pan.*

85g plain flour
30g coconut flour
3 large eggs
240ml milk
120ml water
butter, for frying

Mix the flours together. Make a well in the centre and mix in the eggs, one at a time. Combine the milk and water and add a little at a time to make a thin batter. Put a little butter in a flat frying pan, heat until hot, then swirl it around to make sure the pan is coated. Reduce the heat to moderate and add 2–3 tablespoons of batter. Swirl the batter around so that it coats the bottom of the pan evenly and cook for 2 minutes each side until crisp and slightly browned.

# FLAPJACKS with coconut flour

(MAKES 18–20 SMALL SQUARES)

180g oats
100g wholemeal or spelt flour
160g butter
35g coconut flour
2 tbsp honey or agave
1 tbsp treacle
70g brown sugar
chopped apricots
2 eggs
3–4 tbsp water

Mix together the oats and flours. In a large pan gently melt the butter, honey or agave, treacle and sugar. Stir in the chopped apricots, then fold in the flour mixture. Beat the eggs and add to the mixture. Add water – the mix should be quite moist. Spoon into a square baking tin and bake in a preheated oven at 180°C (gas mark 4) for 15–20 minutes, until lightly browned. Leave to cool in the tin for 5 minutes, then score into squares. Leave to cool and harden in the baking tin before turning out.

# SWEDISH APPLE CAKE with coconut flour

### (MAKE IN A 200MM SQUARE CAKE TIN)

40g coconut flour
135g self-raising white flour
140g sugar
50g flaked almonds
160g butter
70g Truvia
3 eggs
50ml milk
3–4 tart apples, cubed
1 tsp vanilla essence
30ml water

Mix together the coconut and white flours. Generously sprinkle the base of the cake tin with sugar and flaked almonds. Cream the butter and sugar together, add the eggs, milk, vanilla essence and water, sieve in the flour, then fold in the apple cubes. Mix well and tip into the cake tin. Bake in a preheated oven at 180°C (gas mark 4) for 30–40 minutes. Leave to cool in the tin, then turn the cake out and serve upside down.

# APPENDIX 3

## Further Information

**SOME HELPFUL BOOKS**
*Collins Gem GI*, published by HarperCollins. This uses red, amber and green to give information about the GI of hundreds of foods. It also gives many helpful hints about living with a low-GI diet.

*The First Year: Type 2 Diabetes* by Gretchen Becker, published by Robinson. The author, who has Type 2 diabetes, is a sheep farmer who became an expert on diabetes after her own diagnosis. The book is quite technical – not an easy read – and she does not pull her punches about the dire consequences of uncontrolled diabetes, but it is very informative.

*The Diabetes Diet* by Richard K. Bernstein, MD, published by Little, Brown and Co. Diagnosed with diabetes as a child, Dr Bernstein explains why a low- (or no-) carb diet is the diet that people with Type 1 or Type 2 should follow. The book is worth reading even if you decide not to follow such an extreme diet, as it provides a good understanding of the carbohydrate problem.

*In Defence of Food* by Michael Pollan, published by Penguin. A small, easy to read book that examines the way we have been advised to replace good nutritious food with food that is, in the author's opinion, actually bad for us.

*Nourishing Traditions: The Cookbook That Challenges Politically Correct Nutrition and the Diet Dictocrats* by Sally Fallon with Mary G. Enig, published by New Trends Publishing. A big book of 660 pages. The first seventy pages examine the evidence that saturated fat is the cause of modern illness, then argues that saturated fat is necessary for human health and well-being (technical and quite hard to follow). The rest of the book contains information about recent food research, anecdotal evidence and recipes.

*Grain Brain: The Surprising Truth about Wheat, Carbs, and Sugar – Your Brain's Silent Killers* by Dr David Perlmutter, published by Yellow Kite. Dr Perlmutter is both a famous neurologist and a nutritionist who believes that gluten is a dangerous inflammatory protein, responsible for many disorders and illnesses.

## SOME HELPFUL WEBSITES

http://www.patient.co.uk/health/type-2-diabetes: Gives detailed information about Type 2 diabetes.

www.glycemicindex.com/faqsList.php: A website from the University of Sydney containing frequently asked questions and full answers about the glycaemic index and glycaemic load.

www.dietandfitnesstoday.com/glycemicIndexList: A chart giving the GI and GL values (often average values) of a vast number of foods.

www.authoritynutrition.com/foods: An 'evidence based' website that highlights the nutritional benefits of common foods.

http://health.howstuffworks.com/wellness/food-nutrition/facts/the-health-benefits-of-vinegar3.htm: Explains the health benefits of vinegar. This is particularly relevant to people with Type 2 diabetes as vinegar can significantly reduce the glycaemic response to food.

www.uk.lifestyle.yahoo.com/blogs/rachael-anne-hill/butter-margarine-better: Presents the butter versus margarine facts simply and clearly.

www.perthdietclinic.com.au/recipe: The Perth Diet Clinic offers an extensive range of recipes, most of them low fat and low GI.

www.diabetes.org.uk: One of the main diabetes charities in the UK.

# Acknowledgements

My thanks to dietitian Julia Scott Douglas BSc RD SENr DipIOC, who read through the text and answered my many queries and questions.

# Index